Doctors on the Edge

Also by Linden West

Beyond Fragments: Adults, Motivation and Higher Education

Doctors on the Edge

General Practitioners, Health and Learning in the Inner-City

Linden West

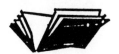

'an association in which the free development of each
is the condition of the free development of all'

FREE ASSOCIATION BOOKS / LONDON / NEW YORK

First published in Great Britain 2001 by
FREE ASSOCIATION BOOKS
57 Warren Street, London W1T 5NR

www.fa-b.com

ISBN 1 85343 522 8 pbk

A CIP catalogue record for this book is available from the British Library.

10 09 08 07 06 05 04 03 02 01
10 9   8   7   6   5   4   3   2   1

Designed and produced for Free Association Books Ltd by
Chase Publishing Services
Printed in the European Union by Athenaeum Press, Gateshead, England

Contents

DEDICATION

For Helen
who taught me about relationships

Preface

This book derives, uniquely, from extensive, in-depth, longitudinal, collaborative and what I term auto/biographical research among twenty-five doctors, more precisely General Practitioners (GPs) or family physicians, working in inner-city contexts. The research focused on the role and well-being of these doctors during a period of changing roles and expectations, including within the management of health care, and at a time of growing concern and criticism over performance and levels of accountability. The inner-city presents its distinct challenges to doctors in the mounting crisis of social exclusion, growing alienation as well as increasing inequalities in health and health care. Put crudely, the poorer you are, the unhealthier you are likely to be and the shorter your life expectancy. The poorer the area in which you live, the more under-resourced and over-stretched are the doctors and services you will use. Doctors as well as patients, in such situations, may often exist on a kind of edge.

Change appears pervasive in health care, as in the wider culture, at many levels and with diverse implications for healing and the professional development of doctors. 'Primary care', or local community-based provision, has moved centre stage and is undergoing yet another reorganisation in which emphasis is given to multi-professional approaches to service delivery, and where professionals have to respond, more directly as well as collaboratively, to national priorities. New systems of appraisal are proposed for doctors, and there are calls for the National Health Service to be managerially more proactive, to ensure that all doctors are up to scratch. For GPs, their independent contractor status – the *sine qua non* of professionalism for some – could eventually give way to an employee/salaried position, as they become direct employees of the Health Service.

Likewise, wider processes of change – part cultural, part political – are impacting on doctors and their work. Relationships between users of services and providers are under constant scrutiny and subject to intense debate in a less deferential, better-educated and more litigious culture. The cultural diversity of the inner-city and the changing status of minority groups – as assimilation gives way to a new politics of difference – has its impact too. The doctor, in such circumstances, requires a cultural sensitivity as well as medical literacy, given the potentially varied meanings of health and well-being across different groups. Moreover, there are various 'postmodern' challenges for the doctor to face including the burgeoning alternative and complementary medicine movements as opposition to the medical model's 'technoculture' and drugs-based treatments.

This book chronicles and theorises, via the stories GPs tell, the impact of social and cultural change on a diverse group of doctors: men and women, black and white, new and long-standing, single-handers and those working in group practices. It documents their many doubts and anxieties about the adequacy of initial and continued learning, and the bio-medical model, in the face of patients' complex experiences and pathologies and their own responses to them. It explores the psychological and emotional distress many GPs experience, and the difficulties of addressing this in a medical culture in which doctors are often, or so it seems, supposed to cope in splendid isolation. However, the book also offers many examples of highly eclectic and imaginative responses to challenging times, and to what is involved in becoming a more effective and reflective practitioner. This is to be understood in psychological and cultural as well as medical terms. It is, in part, about engaging with and learning from the diversity of self, as a basis for engaging with and better connecting with the diversity of others.

The book details the stories of doctors who, because of their own multiple identities and experiences of oppression, have often felt on the margins of their profession. Such doctors – 'outsider-insiders' – raise radical questions about the health of medicine. These include concerns about the adequacy of their initial training and the patriarchal, individualistic and, at times, emotionally immature professional world they inhabit. At the cutting edge of biographical reappraisal and experiment, these narratives tell of learning to be more authentic doctors, as well as emotionally literate subjects, often despite rather than because of the system.

Certain doctors cope better than others with the stresses of their work in a context of uncertain change and the pressure of the city. Some are more open to the developmental possibilities of the postmodern moment, including what may be a crisis in scientific medicine and its positivist assumptions. Some are more anxious about the future and their capacity to adapt in changing times; yet others remain haunted by particular 'failures'. Some, especially Asian single-handers, talk of racism and of being scapegoated in what seems, at times, more of a blaming than a learning culture. These issues take us into the territory of cultural psychology, which lies at the interpretive heart of the book. As do the stories from a number of female doctors, who explored their deeply gendered lives, and workplaces, in which caring and emotional labour remains predominantly 'women's work'.

The book constitutes a substantial challenge to some of the cultural norms of the medical world, not least the myth of omnipotence: a doctor must always know best, and cope, like 'good men should'. Some GPs offer an alternative vision and practice: of greater emotional openness and honest communication across the profession and the willingness to learn from and work with patients and their stories, as well as colleagues in ancillary professions. This book also chronicles the courage involved in learning autobiographically; not only from patients but also from the 'patient' within.

Acknowledgments

This project has taken five years to complete, from inception to finishing the book. It has been a highly significant learning process, which includes greater understanding of others as well as of self. The project would have been impossible without particular people and the help, support, encouragement and guidance they have provided. A book is always and inevitably a product of many and diverse people: in a quite fundamental sense, writing and research are a collective process, as we draw on others, and their stories, to give meaning and shape to our own. Despite the individualism that pervades academic culture, ideas are social in nature, nurtured in relationship and in a range of 'invisible colleges': those networks of people to which we belong and from which we draw inspiration and nourishment. When I write, I know others are there with me, supporting, cajoling as well as questioning my words. 'Doctors on the Edge' is but one contribution to a conversation with many authors.

The 'networks' include the twenty-five doctors whose stories taught me much about healing, lifelong learning as well as of courage and integrity in difficult times. I hope they consider their effort has been worthwhile, and feel I have done justice to the complexity of all they shared with me. I apologise to those whose material is not used explicitly, but they are there, informing the text in many ways. In fact all the doctors remain with me, in a psychological sense, sustaining a faith in, and a vision of, the possibilities for lifelong learning and a more humane, socially aware and psychologically literate medical profession in changing times. Many of these doctors are at the cutting edge of all that is good and life enhancing in their profession.

I would wish to express thanks to many close friends, especially Helen Reynolds, my partner, whose love and support made the research possible; to Wilma Fraser, a soul mate, and someone who, in Adrienne Rich's words, has gone 'the hard way' with me. I would also like to thank Jonny Burton, whose wisdom, enthusiasm and friendship are greatly valued. Wilma, Jonny and Helen read a draft of the book, and made many valuable suggestions. Thanks are also due to Steve Wakelam, for advice on the structure and style of the book, and for the encouragement to experiment as a writer; to Nod Miller, whose support and encouragement have been invaluable, over many years. Also to Nick Riding for conversations, on countless training runs, about, believe it or not, gender and the nature of psychoanalysis, and of what it means to be a man.

Thanks also to members of the Innovations in Education and Research Group – to Jonny Burton again, Penny Morris, Kathy Burton, Mike Carmi, Alex Jamieson, Madeleine Reiss, Steve Hiew and Vicki Souster – who offered support and experience, in a caring way, over a long period. I would also wish to thank colleagues in the Medway Medical Educators Group, including Ann Richmond, Nathan Nathan, Om Singh, Awadh Jha, Peter Green and Ann Douse, for their enthusiasm and practical suggestions as to how to establish the project in the Medway Towns.

Similarly thanks are due to colleagues in university continuing education and the SCUTREA network (Standing Conference of University Teachers and Researchers in the Education of Adults) particularly Cheryl Hunt, who helped me rediscover the spiritual in learning; to Richard Edwards, for many stimulating ideas; to Bill Williamson and John Field, for their encouragement at a difficult personal time. And to Agnieszka Bron and others in the European Society for Research into the Education of Adults, especially members of the Life Histories/Biographies Research Group. Agnieszka is a source of constant inspiration, partly because she has the gift, like all good teachers, of making critical suggestions in positive ways. Thanks also to a number of old and dear friends including Colin Kirkwood, Francis Beckett and Malcolm Clarke; to Jill Halpen, a guiding light; and to Carolyn Jongeward and Tony Lockhart, whose struggles touched my own, and helped me in my journey.

Last but never least, thanks to Mary Calthrop, Eve Burr and Marisol Menendez who provided patient administrative support to the project as well as to Thames Postgraduate Medical and Dental Education who provided resources for some of the research. And to Trevor Brown, from Free Association Books, and all his colleagues, for supporting the proposal, and who remained patient as the deadline passed, and the manuscript remained undelivered.

Please note that permission has been sought for all copyright material reproduced herein. Thanks to Arcadia Books, and to John Berger, for permission to quote from John Berger and Jean Mohr's *A Fortunate Man*; to the University of Chicago Press for allowing me to use a quote from the second edition of Hannah Arendt's *The Human Condition*; to Oxford University Press for material from Herbert Grierson's *Donne, Poetical Works*; to Berg Publishers in Oxford for permission to quote from Simon Sinclair's book, *Making Doctors* and to Routledge for the use of material from Andrew Samuel's *The Political Psyche*.

Linden West
Canterbury, England

1

On the Edge of Story

Landscapes can be deceptive. Sometimes a landscape seems to be less a setting for the life of its inhabitants than a curtain behind which their struggles, achievements and accidents take place ... landmarks are no longer only geographic but also biographic and personal ... [Dr John Sassall] began to realise that he must face his own imagination, even explore it. It must no longer lead always to the 'unimaginable', as it had with the Master Mariners contemplating the possible fury of the elements – or, as in his case, to his contemplating only fights with the jaws of death itself ... He began to realise that imagination had to be lived with on every level: his own imagination first – because otherwise this could distort his observation – and then the imagination of his patients.

J. Berger and J. Mohr, *A Fortunate Man*

Diagnosis ... becomes problematic ... when working with diverse communities, in the inner-city or with refugees. Someone who stays at home and looks after a parent: is this separation anxiety or taking responsibility for older people? Is not looking a person in the eye about culture or avoidance? And people who go on endlessly about the body but not the mind, is this a real psychological problem or a non-western, non-dualistic alternative?

D. Ingleby, 'Culture and Medical Health: A Radical Agenda'

Introduction: Of and About Stories

This is a book of and about stories: stories that doctors tell of their work, their patients and themselves in difficult and demanding social contexts, and during a time of major change and widespread uncertainty in health care and medicine. It tells too of the professional culture doctors inhabit and what facilitates or inhibits their well-being and professional development, including the role of initial training and what has come to be termed 'lifelong learning'. The book also encompasses stories concerning the professional and private interface in doctors' lives, and how the personal interconnects, for better or worse, with the public role. It includes what tends to be omitted when doctors tell stories, particularly under the gaze of critical politicians, health service managers, or their colleagues. There is a focus too on the role of story itself and its potential importance in meaning-making and psychological well-being

1

in a culture in flux, where some of the big stories of 'modernity' – about the role of science in medicine, for instance – are fiercely contested.

Human beings, as Jerome Bruner observed (1990), do not terminate at their own skin, they are, for better or worse, embodiments of a culture, selecting from among its symbols and discourses, consciously or otherwise, what to believe and what to say. Culture and history are played out in individual biographies, narrowing or increasing options for personal or collective experiment. Biographies reflect the play of history in particular lives and in specific times, of what seems possible and what may be silenced or repressed. Biographies, however, can also serve as sites for resistance and radical opposition to myths which have outlived their usefulness, and for challenging what powerful others might say and wish us to believe. We are all influenced by context and social affiliation, by what is easy or not easy to articulate in specific contexts and power relationships, by what is considered respectable on the part of peers and significant others (West, 1996). This applies no less in medicine than in other sub-cultures and this book raises major issues about the relationship between dominant stories within medical culture, and those that tend to be marginalised and even silenced altogether. Some stories matter more than others, and particular experiences may be difficult, even dangerous, to articulate to self, let alone to colleagues. The relationship between representation (the story) and reality (experience) is far from simple and linear. Stories, as Foucault and others have taught (Foucault, 1979; White and Epston, 1990) 'constitute' as well as 'reflect' experience: reality and representation are not easily prised apart. Doctors, as this book reveals, are no exception. They may be induced, consciously or unconsciously, to construct stories about their work according to particular regimes of truth. Careers and status may depend on it. But in this postmodern moment, 'history' may be creating more space for diverse and even subversive stories of doctors and their work.

On the Edge of the Profession

This book focuses on General Practitioners (GPs) and it is relevant that they have been, historically at least, situated on the edge of the medical profession, at the interface between the 'scientific' claims of mainstream medicine, and the messy swamp of actual lives and uncertain symptoms (Schon, 1987). The 'problem' in any consultation for the GP – interpreting the patient and her story and responding appropriately – raises questions which are part social, part cultural, part psychic, part organic, part spiritual, part existential, and, in part, to do with the here and now of the doctor–patient relationship. The hardest task can be to define what the problem actually is, let alone prescribe a solution, including, for some doctors, encouraging patients to articulate more of their own stories. By the time the patient sees the specialist, a degree of clarification, a narrowing of possibilities will have occurred. GPs are, frequently and increasingly, a first port of call for many isolated, vulnerable people in distressed communities. GPs, by definition, are generalists, 'Jacks of all trades', in a profession where specialist, hard, 'scientific' knowledge has traditionally counted most. Reid (1982), among others, has described their frequent alienation from the medical mainstream and they can feel marginal in medical school, while academic General Practice, as McWhinney (1996) notes, in its attempts to discover a distinct epistemological basis, fits uncomfortably in the highly scientist milieu of the medical school and the wider academy. General Practice, in this, and other respects, is under constant pressure to become more 'scientific', (i.e. less pragmatic and 'soft'), as well as more theoretical and quantitative. The trends, and tensions, are paradoxical in what is highly contested space.

Fortunate Men, and Women?

John Berger and Jean Mohr's story of Doctor John Sassall, who worked as a General Practitioner (GP) in a poor, deprived rural community, was an important influence in the development of this book. They spent time with a doctor, encouraging him to tell and reflect on his story and its diverse meanings. The insights generated shaped many of the themes explored, in-depth, and at length, with twenty-five GPs who worked in the different environment of the inner-city. (This is the setting, although we shall see that issues to do with poverty or powerlessness have striking similarities whether the setting is urban or rural.) John Sassall was faced, most days, with the consequences of material poverty and the perpetual struggle, for many of his patients, to eke a living from limited and fragile resources. He faced the despair of oppressed people and a distress which was often more socio-cultural than medical in origin. He talked of 'obstinacy and prejudice', born of that defeat and despair and of the poverty of the imagination which can compound oppression. Sassall's narrative is forged from the need to come to terms with the power of his own imagination and the impact of others' stories. Some of his themes apply equally to so many doctors working in the fragile and fragmented townscape of the inner-city.

Berger and Mohr focused, in part, on the social interactions between a doctor and his patients, and the cultural norms and expectations that shaped them. They wanted to understand better the doctor's responses to people and their suffering, including what was triggered, in Sassall's own self and imagination, by particular patients and specific encounters. They explored his interpretation and negotiation of such experience, including his coping with feelings of frustration, ignorance, uncertainty and, at times, impotence as a doctor. In so doing, Berger and Mohr captured some of the sense of inadequacy and futility which can haunt a doctor. They laid bare some of the complex biographical topography normally hidden behind professional insouciance. They revealed some of the personal struggle involved in seeking to be an authentic and effective doctor beyond the blandishments of government and managerial policy pronouncements.

Their book may be read, in more contemporary terms, as a chronicle of a 'lifelong learner', not in any narrow utilitarian sense, but in profounder ways; in the human struggles, which we all share, to create insight and meaning from the diverse fragments of confused experience. And, like the good novelist, in the struggle to transform some of the chaos and complexities of this experience into a more meaningful whole: an act of artistry, heart, moral courage, imagination and intellect (Randall, 1995; West, 1996). Sassall embarked, in fact, on a complex journey of self and emotional understanding, reading Freud and attempting, albeit alone, to analyse his own character traits, and their roots in past and present relationships. He attempted to confront his demons, and those of his patients. More prosaically, he sought, constantly, to improve standards of care. He worked hard on his skills and knowledge base and invested in a range of new technologies. He read all the journals, attended postgraduate lectures at a local hospital and sought to ground his consultations in the latest research. He practised 'evidence-based medicine' long before the term was in use as common currency.

Yet, despite his commitment to learning and professional development, Sassall found no lasting peace or sustained satisfaction. Like too many other doctors, he committed suicide. Berger and Mohr's study details frequent bouts of depression and the restless, often unrequited quest for 'answers', and for meaning, in his work and wider life. He was ultra-sensitive to his shortcomings, to the messiness of the role and the uncertainties surrounding the nature and causes of ill-health. He felt guilty about setbacks, becoming, in consequence, more susceptible to the suffering of others. Suffering, as it were, posed questions about the value of the moment, and raised issues about the emptiness of his own life. If he was, in certain respects, 'a fortunate man' doing what he wanted, pursuing what he wished, with relative social status and material security, he struggled and suffered too. His inner landscape must, at times, have seemed as bleak as those of some of his patients.

Dr David Widgery worked in the somewhat different townscape of the East End of London. He died in tragic circumstances and was suffering a deep depression at the time. His autobiography (Widgery, 1993), provides a powerful commentary on the waste of many lives in the inner-city, and the effects on a doctor's emotional health. David describes, at one point, visiting the flat of a man who had been depressed and had finally drunk himself to death. The dead man had been there for six days 'rotting on a vast mound of empties' and the smell was 'rich and sickly'. David also wrote about the good and rewarding aspects of the work: of visiting a couple, Mr and Mrs Foley, he an ex-docker with a history of active trade unionism, she a loyal wife. Mr Foley was dying from cancer and David recalled getting to know the family well and, in the process, discovering more of Mr Foley's involvement in trade union struggles in the docks; music to David's Marxist ears. David gave time to the Foleys, enabling them to tell more of their story, when it really mattered. Perhaps he found it difficult to share the complexities of his own story, including a crisis of faith, when it mattered most. David wrote of feeling over-whelmed by the waste, neglect and hopelessness of parts of the East End:

> ... the grinding down of the optimism with which I came to the East End nearly twenty years ago, into a kind of grudging weariness punctuated with bouts of petty fury. When I came here ... I didn't know what the bruised face of a heroin addict was like, or how children could be locked up, four in a room, by a drunken father as punishment ... And now I do. I know what decomposed bodies of alcoholics smell like after two weeks ...
> ... my experience reflects a much larger loss of hope, morale and optimism ... I'm watching something die and I wish I wasn't. Perhaps the best thing that can be done is to record the process.

He chronicled what he perceived to be an East End culture savaged by economic and social forces and the individualistic illusions and nihilism of capitalist consumerism. His book is a record of growing disenchantment with the doctor's role, in the light of a ubiquitous social pathology, and with the direction many colleagues seemed to be taking: 'the New Model GP' hunched over the computer screen calculating uptake and turnover, 'auditing not clinical skill but fiscal returns'. Businessmen rather than clinicians or healers.

Disillusionment can be the lot of many doctors. An increasing number are reported as suffering from severe stress, clinical depression, alcoholism; and more doctors are committing suicide (RCGP, 1994). There is accumulating evidence of declining morale, increased turnover and intense problems of recruitment and retention, especially among GPs in the inner-city (McBride and Metcalfe1995; Rout, 1996; Bennet, 1998). Such data raise basic questions at the heart of the present study: about the GP's changing role and how this is best managed, about how particular doctors cope in the harsh townscape of the inner-city, and about the role and parameters of initial and lifelong learning, including the extent to which doctors are enabled to understand and manage the psychological and cultural dimensions of their work. Questions also arise about the health of the medical sub-culture itself. This is the territory of cultural psychology, and of being a GP in the inner-city.

A starting point for the study, in the case of ten of the doctors, was an expe-riential or self-directed learning project, established under the auspices of 'The London Implementation Zone Educational Initiative' or LIZEI, in the mid-

1990s. LIZEI was a response to the Tomlinson Review of hospital and primary care services in inner-London (Tomlinson, 1992), which suggested that General Practice was often of dubious quality and grossly under-resourced. LIZEI sought to 'recruit, retain and refresh' GPs in such areas (Carmi and Hiew, 1997). The aim was to improve standards as well as support hard-pressed doctors, especially (but not exclusively) the large number of 'ethnic', 'single-handers' who had gone to the areas others tended to avoid. LIZEI tried, as detailed in Chapter 4, to combine a political and managerialist agenda to improve standards with a bottom–up approach to professional development and the continuing education of GPs.

In 1996 I was asked to evaluate the impact of one self-directed learning programme (SDL), as perceived by participants themselves. The idea was to use largely unstructured and confidential interviews, and a collaborative approach to their interpretation, to establish what doctors really thought and felt about such learning, and its impact, in changing times. Over a period, and with the support of the original group and the recruitment of others, the study developed into a comprehensive, in-depth and collaborative analysis of diverse aspects of the role, including its autobiographical and psychological dimensions. The research was intended to encompass the nature of healing as well as learning; the relationship between the personal and professional in doctors' lives; and the complex interplay of a doctor's identity – whether as a man, a woman, Asian or gay, for instance – with those of patients.

Starting Points

I want to begin the story with some initial glimpses into the lifeworlds of particular GPs, gleaned from early interviews, which motivated me to explore issues in greater depth and over time. Glimpses, for instance, of the inner-city and its challenges. Dr Claire Barker (all names, as explained in Chapter 3, are pseudonyms and specific locations, and some details, have been changed to preserve anonymity), works in London. She had recently moved from a practice in a deprived area, to a surgery in a less demanding part of town. She described the practice she was leaving:

> ... It was in a very poor area ... poor in terms of not having really any money at all. And you go into the house and it has got the classic large television set and probably very little else ... There is ... the council estate area and high unemployment, large families, and not much money and also very poor support really for the patients generally. Very demanding patients. One of the things I found very difficult it is difficult to make eye contact with them. You would go and do visits at home. You would have to ask them to

call the dog off you, which was normally a great big dog and I like dogs, but not great big dogs when I am working. And you have to say would you mind turning the television off and that didn't normally go down too well. Sometimes I was too frightened to ask them to turn the television off and also you went in and Dad would be playing computer games and would sort of say 'she's 'ere' and that would be that really.

... I mean Hackney is known to be a very poor area and again poverty brings its own problems in dealing with the patients and it takes a very special person, I think, to be able to deal with that. I could do it in the short term, the idea of having to do those battles for twenty-five years because one of the most important things in general practice is to be able to communicate with your patients and if you can't get over that initial level of communication, if you can't make eye contact and you can't communicate, and also I don't like confrontation and I don't like aggression and when people tell me to fuck off on the phone, for no obvious reason, I don't like it.

... It is not so much the patients who come up to the consulting room, normally I feel fairly safe. We have a panic button, there are other people around. But going out and visiting people, even during daylight hours, on my own, I feel very vulnerable. I have got an obvious doctor's bag. I do carry controlled drugs because if somebody has a myocardial ... I need to be able to treat them appropriately and so you are obviously fairly vulnerable if you do a daytime visit in an area like that. It is obvious that you are the doctor and going into people's houses when you are not made to feel welcome and there is a level of aggression before you have said anything. Also I found that a lot of the people sort of felt that it was their right, it is my right to have a doctor, and it made me begin to feel like saying – well actually I am a human being ...

Claire described services on a particular estate:

For instance ... the psychiatric services there, well the child psychiatry services, to get your child seen to, the child has either had to threaten to kill someone else, threaten to kill themselves, or have been expelled from school for five days. One day is not sufficient, it has got to be a five-day expulsion. Otherwise forget it and this is the most needy of populations. Yet because it is such an awful area people don't want to work there, myself included, so they find it very difficult to attract both the GPs, and the psychiatrists, and all the other people, health visitors. So in an area where they really need the input it is very difficult to keep the health care professionals, simply because you are constantly so stretched, emotionally as well as work-wise ... I had a lady who had had twins and she said 'well I feel like throwing them out the window'.

... Well I have to say that just about everyone was on anti-depressants ... I mean the depression was just mammoth and I am not surprised they were depressed. The lives they were living I think I would have been depressed. It was certainly a bolt from the blue for most of them. No money, being abused by at least one relative, dreadful lives, dreadful lives. And whatever people say about money doesn't matter and you can have a good life if you are poor, I have actually come to the conclusion that it does matter and it is much easier to have a good life if you have got money. Money doesn't buy happiness but it makes it much more comfortable to enjoy your life if you don't have to worry about doing the shop in Tesco's and whether you can buy shoes for the children and never being able to go out ...

Diagnosis can be problematic in the inner-city. Dr Jane Kelly described a particular patient:

... she is a hugely obese lady with hiatus hernia and arthritis because of her weight, a bit of asthma, lots of pain mainly because of her weight. And the medical approach to that would be to try and get her to diet, which is a losing battle, prescribe her pain killers, prescribe her something for her hiatus hernia, provide creams for her rashes and then leave it at that. You have provided what you as a doctor are able to provide. Over the years that I have known her and perhaps because I take a different approach, what has actually been revealed is that she was sexually abused from ten to sixteen by her brother and raped by her cousins and has an incredibly low self-esteem, absolutely consumed with guilt and therefore self-destructive. She self-mutilates as well, which she doesn't often show or presents as sort of skin problems that are actually a product of her self-mutilation. Can't comply with a diet because eating is part of her sort of self-destruction if you like and you know needs that sorting out. Doesn't need me filling her up with drugs and referring her to more and more specialists. So that, you know, I could be a doctor that had just accepted the things she presents. She has never presented the sexual abuse. It has come out because I have teased it out of her I suppose. So that is the two sides of it. She could go to one doctor and go away with a load of pills. I don't say that I have got her any more sorted out because I have been struggling to find some sort of appropriate coun-selling, but she has opened up and she has talked to me and she has not talked to anybody else and it is a start of her healing really. I wouldn't be creating any healing by just filling her up with tablets.

Shades of Diversity

The challenging implications of cultural diversity in the inner-city, for doctors as well as in relationship with patients, were early themes. John Chan worked in Tottenham:

> ... On our patient list we have about a third who are refugees from northern Iraq, eastern Turkey, that sort of thing, so we have got two translators, interpreters who work here, not quite full time, but near enough. They work here every day of the week. You have probably noticed on the walls a lot of notices in Turkish for that reason, so that has sort of skewed the sort of practice that you see now ...

John mentioned a case of a young, female refugee:

> ... she's married, they tend to marry quite young, not bad looking and she always comes in looking reasonably pleasant ... and she has actually been with us for two or three years now, she has a council flat, wasn't moved from one place to another, so she is lucky and settled, got her money because either she was working or she claimed Social Security or whatever and she used to get all these migraines, headaches, aches and pains in the neck. And in the end because it clearly wasn't a physical illness, she had some form of mild depression and we thought it was due to her being a refugee, being on the move, and away from her family, and so we asked these questions – 'have you got family there?' They do have family there. 'Do you worry about them?' 'Oh yes we worry about them.' 'Do you ring them often?' 'We can't afford to ring them often'; and in a way we kind of constructed a history for her by asking her leading questions and this went on for a year or two, not quite knowing why she didn't get better – 'surely you are settled here now, got friends, got money, bought a little car' and then one day she came up and said 'I am really in big trouble now.' She was actually full of tears and it transpired that she had been childless in a five-year marriage and being childless meant being possessed by evil, unclean, useless, not a real woman and the mother-in-law saying 'We are going to throw you out of the window if you don't bring us a child tomorrow morning.' And that was what was causing all these headaches, all this time, but she was so ashamed of it she couldn't even see a doctor about it.
> ... We actually found a Turkish-speaking doctor who, for all kinds of reasons, was unemployed as a doctor, OK, and he was actually working part time on some refugee project with the local health authority. So we got him to do some of these counselling sessions, a few here, and a few people got very attached to him. Most of them still just came back ...

Some of the patients, as it turned out, were Kurds and resented, for obvious reasons, being counselled by a Turk. Life on the front line, somewhere in inner-London.

An Outsider, Among Outsiders

Dr Aidene Croft talked, early on, of being a GP and of her own problems. And she introduced important aspects of her identity:

> ... I've recently become a single-handed GP having broken away from the group practice which is now two partners and used to be three ... Well the short answer is I was asked to leave the group practice due to a dispute ... I feel it was directly related to the pressures on general practice ... Administrative burden, pay ... The co-op [a doctors' co-operative] has made a big difference to me, but not having the co-op would be an ongoing nightmare, I'm thinking of other GPs. And reaccreditation is not pleasant to think about in the future, and things that get in the way of actually talking to patients, which is a lot of this evidence-based medicine. And working to guidelines and pressures to be a robot, really, a technician for what the government believes to be a cost-effective service ...
>
> ... I became ill and it left major problems for the rest of ... the remaining doctors that was compounded by the fact that financial issues came into it. But I don't think the communication would have broken down had there not been the degree of strain and stress, so I think it was a direct corollary of the stress ... Yes, the kind of stress ... of providing services, when so much of hospital services are being 'dumped', in inverted commas, on GPs, when the patient expectations have increased, when the administrative burdens have been increased, when the expenses have increased and then on top of all that a doctor becomes sick ... what has been burdensome then becomes an intolerable burden and I feel that that was reflected in the breakdown in communication ... feeling unsupported in the health service ... And all this reaccreditation, I just turn the page, I can't be doing with it. If they come to reaccredit me, I'll ... I was just going to say 'I'll just leave.' I mean working with the government breathing down one shoulder, the RCGP [Royal College of General Practitioners] – our pillory tower of ivory – breathing down another, and somebody with reaccreditation breathing down the third shoulder if you had one, it's a nightmare! ... I think the 'oughts' should be how do we keep our patients safe, protect their health for the future and treat the symptoms that they present us with. It's terribly difficult because I can also see the point of evidence-based medicine. You know if you don't have good evidence well don't medicalise people. You know I think Western medicine has created dependence so that they can no longer manage the

simplest medical problem, not to mention a crisis, without referring to the doctor. So I think this culture has created a really difficult situation for people because they don't know what they ought to come to the doctor with. Do they come to the doctor in the first hour of the fever because it might be meningitis? When do they come ... the general public is completely confused.

... I mean I had to get ill last year, quite ill ... family demands. You know, if you actually have to be elsewhere, then you have to stop. I think if I were on my own and there wasn't a stop that I had to make I think I would probably be a workaholic, which isn't good for anybody's health. Within the last year I've phoned Samaritans, I've phoned the BMA Stress Line. It's not been a typical year. I mean I would hope that not every year I would have the amount of stress to do with group practice disputes; I've had the BMA Industrial Relations Officer, I've seen the HFSA Medical Advisor, I've seen the LMC Representative. I've used all of those sources of support. So one way I do it is by identifying the support and using it. I've had legal advice through friends. But on the everyday ... it's been an extraordinary year. I've relied on previous experience ... my family, I would say ... and the other people that I work with here. Yes, they are a nice bunch of people to work with.

... I'm in a lesbian relationship, but that's generally known within my immediate vicinity and even within a larger – it's not something that worries me – in fact I think I'd probably be glad to be a representative: against the assumption that everybody is straight, while not particularly wanting to have it blazoned on every street corner or whatever. But there are a lot of lesbian practitioners in London, so if one of them has a voice again I don't think it is a particularly unique voice, but the voice is there and the assumption shouldn't be made ... I don't know whether there are other gay doctors that are part of your research.

Aidene decided, after some initial hesitation, to participate in the longer-term study. She was an outsider who often felt uncomfortable within, as well as sceptical towards, what was sometimes a very 'laddish medical culture'.

A Sort of Madness

Daniel Cohen also introduced a crisis in his career in his first interview:

Yes, I had been in the job for ten or eleven years, full time, which meant nine sessions a week, that is nine surgeries a week, each with maybe twenty patients. I wasn't doing any post-graduate education, either receiving it or giving it. I wasn't doing any research. I didn't have adequate time for reflection. I was doing lots of on-call and I was knackered and at one stage I got ill, I had a heart problem in 1989 ... Well all the NHS changes, with all their negative aspects....

General Practice, he said, was:

... like swimming along an endless river and trying to have intelligent conversations while you are swimming. There is very little of the time that I delude myself that I am treating people, or curing people, or making dramatic interventions but I think I am in the river with them rather than watching them from the bank. But I am hoping that my head may be a few inches higher above the water than theirs at times, no doubt there are also times when their heads are rather higher above the water than mine. But at least you're having conversations as you swim along that are hopefully making their lives a little more comfortable and a little more intelligible.

... I don't think that I personally can ever get away from the feeling of intense frustration and often exasperation with that [limited time]. I doubt if I ever go a week and probably I don't ever go a day without thinking this is totally insane and nobody should be doing this, to have twenty-five patients in the course of one morning bursting through that bloody door one after the other with problems, each of which would floor an experienced psychiatrist, clinical psychologist. I regularly have the thought that this is mad and I am going and am giving up. So it is real roller coaster, but what I think keeps me going is another sort of dialogue which I also have with myself, which says something like 'This is a miraculous facility that this country, in spite of all its flaws, has a service where anybody can walk through the door of a trained professional bringing problems of body or mind or soul and get some time for it and occasionally something happens, or more than occasionally something happens, which really makes the difference.' And that is hugely worth preserving. It doesn't exist in most other countries and there is no other profession in this country to whom people have open access to take those sorts of issues.

We were to spend three years together considering some of 'the madness', and how he finally transcended the crisis of mid-career. We reflected, in dialogue, on the range of factors – including therapy, learning, intimate relationships, becoming an educator, the culture of the practice in which he worked and relationships with colleagues, as well as his Jewish identity and a burgeoning spirituality – in his emerging biography and the part each played in recomposing and reinvigorating a career. We considered together, at length, the gendered nature of being a doctor and a man, and how gender was presently in uncertain flux, symbolically and in actual lived relationships, and the opportunities such times presented.

Daniel and all the doctors considered the shifting, uncertain parameters of health and illness in the inner-city, and in transitional times. Their stories are set in contexts of constant change in health care, and of intense and critical scrutiny of the doctor's role and performance. The stories draw back the curtains and illuminate a highly gendered world, a world in which a struggle is unfolding between competing discourses about the knowledge required to be a doctor, and the relative importance of psychological, intuitive and narrative ways of knowing, as well as cultural literacy, alongside medical science.

Structure of the Book

Before turning to these stories, I locate them, in the next chapter, within the uncertain context of the British Health Service and a medical culture where doctors have been socialised into believing that they ought to know, and cope, whatever the cost. The stories are also set within a changing, uncertain and anxious society where older, paternalistic structures appear to have broken down. The chapter explains current changes in doctors' relationships with other health-care workers, as well as in the organisation of primary health care; amid the growing emphasis, mainly for economic reasons, on community-based provision. The story is also told of GPs' historically marginal position in a hierarchical profession, where specialists, and speciality, have tended to be deified. And where anthropological/sociological and psychological insights have often, in training and in life, been dismissed or even derided by some of the powers that be. I also develop further the idea of gendered cultural psychology and its role in interpreting and theorising the stories doctors tell.

In Chapter 3 I explain how auto/biographical research derives from the belief that the complex stories of individuals are essential to understanding the dialectics of structure and agency in particular lives (Miller and West, 1998). Moreover auto/biographical research challenges conventional genre distinctions between self and other, memory and present, researcher and researched in interpreting lives and composing texts about them. Martin Buber (1965) has coined a phrase 'imagining the real' in which research is conceived to be a collaborative act of the imagination as much as the intellect, of feeling as well as thought; a shared, empathic recreation and reinterpretation of experience. The use of such methods is unusual in medical research where the gold standard remains experimental procedures and the randomised control trial, even when researching educational experience and its outcomes.

The doctors' narratives are used in three main ways in structuring the book. First, there is a focus on single life stories, which, because of the richness and complexity of the material, illuminate particular themes in poignant ways.

Second, stories are grouped according to one particular theme: such as men managing change. And third, by using a collection of life stories as a source of evidence in supporting the development of an overall argument, such as that concerning the nature of learning and the importance of self-knowledge and cultural literacy in being an effective GP.

Chapter 4, 'Learning in the City', describes 'self-directed learning groups' in parts of inner-London: the starting point, as explained, for the whole study. The chapter reveals how the groups sometimes offered a lifeline for particular doctors, enabling them to explore clinical problems and possibilities in the broadest sense. The chapter evaluates the evidence on the impact of SDL, and its contribution to the development of self-directed learning more widely in London.

Chapter 5, 'A Wet Monday Morning', is a chronicle of how themes that were to become central to the whole study, emerged unpredictably in the stress of a day's surgery. Two doctors were upset when coping with aggressive patients, complaints, management and financial pressures as well as domestic and personal problems, carried over from the weekend. The boundaries of bio-graphical research, between, for instance, research and therapy, can be problematic at such moments while the stories raise the big question about the viability and desirability of GPs as independent contractors: of being a business person, a manager as well as a clinician.

Chapter 6, 'The Cutting Edge', focuses on two doctors who transcended, in part, crises in careers and personal lives. Daniel Cohen used education, personal therapy and a close relationship to recompose a more integrated pro-fessional, personal and cultural identity. Aidene Croft is a lesbian who, as indicated, never accepted 'malestream', patriarchal and 'laddish assumptions'. Both doctors can be considered as outsiders on the inside of a professional world. The chapter illustrates how being on such a cultural edge can stimulate an eclectic and authentic engagement with alternative perspectives, including psychotherapy, complementary therapies and narrative-based medicine.

Chapter 7 considers the stories of three women GPs with childcare respon-sibilities. The chapter details their struggles to hold professional as well as personal selves together, and the psychological cost to them. But these are also times where gendered relationships are being questioned, and where some individual men and women are renegotiating and sharing roles in more personally authentic ways.

Chapter 8, 'Men Behaving Sadly', focuses on three male GPs struggling with changing roles, uncertain beliefs and selves. There is a story of a doctor in mid-career crisis, which includes needing to resolve a range of unfulfilled ambitions and 'failures'. Another doctor is sad about the state of the profession and the fact that his counselling skills and Balint training have an uncertain place in the 'five minute culture'. The third story comes from an overseas doctor who was expected to achieve in a family of high achievers. He felt a failure in 'the backwater of general practice'.

Chapter 9, ' Cultures of Silence', illustrates how hard, even dangerous, it can be for doctors to admit to psychological problems, and how particular doctors may hide core aspects of an identity – such as their sexuality – even from experiential groups specifically designed to explore the impact of patients on doctors, and where sexuality may be an important factor in the relationship.

Chapter 10, 'Performance and Underperformance' provides two contrasting case studies in 'failure', including seeking to resurrect a run-down practice and failing to deal with a badly performing colleague.

Chapter 11 considers the narratives of doctors from minority ethnic backgrounds, working in much derided single-handed practices; it illustrates how racism and being scapegoated can sour a professional life and inhibit lifelong learning.

In Chapter 12, a doctor actively engaged in the politics of health care offers an analysis of the crisis of general practice, and how this brings into question the independent contractor status of the GP. The chapter also illustrates, at a different level, how men's stories are often constructed around public roles and performance; but how collaborative research can transcend such norms, allowing a shared exploration of the emotional price of public performance.

In the final chapter, on the basis of these narratives, I consider the health of a deeply gendered world, but also how what has been thought marginal may be central to becoming a more effective doctor. How the physician as healer may be about to rise, phoenix-like, as a counter-balance to the impersonality of modern medicine. Cultural and psychological literacies, including autobiographical awareness, are in fact essential to understanding and connecting with the 'otherness' of the patient in the consulting room. The book concludes with a challenge: that the evidence of distress and depression among many doctors is, in part, a consequence of a rigid culture in which emotions are often frightening, and where it is, too frequently, hard to talk and to learn.

2
A Gendered Cultural Psychology in
Transitional Times

... We cannot be comfortable with the mechanical metaphor which dominates medicine, or with the mind/body dualism derived from it ... the value we place on relationships influences our valuation of knowledge. Those who value relationships tend to know the world by experience rather than what Charles Taylor calls 'instrumental' and 'disengaged' reason. Experience engages our feelings as well as our intellect. The emotions play a very significant part in general practice, and ... are seriously neglected in medicine as a whole.

James McWhinney, 'The Importance of Being Different'

Every effort is made to protect doctors from the public, rather than the other way round ... This notably open-minded approach to medical misconduct ensures that no hard-working, conscientious professional will be suspended or lose his job for something trivial. Such as being disrespectful or rude to patients. Or insensitive or bullying. Even for showing outright contempt. There seems little point in any of us complaining about a consultant obstetrician [who] blamed women themselves for misunderstandings about hormone replacement therapy ... 'Women do not think like men' [he insisted]. 'Men do not rely on friends, next-door neighbours or relatives for medical advice or information; they go looking for the written word' ...

Catherine Bennett, 'Dirty Doctors'

Introduction

In this chapter I locate GPs and their work within the wider context of a growing challenge to the medical profession and its performance. Levels of competence are being questioned, and this includes seeking to address the problem of poorly performing doctors against mounting criticism of what is often derided as 'cosy' self-regulation. The current position of GPs has also to be located within the rapidly shifting scenery of changing roles and changing organisations, in which the old-style family doctor is considered, by some, to be redundant. I also introduce the conceptual frame underpinning the study: what I term a gendered cultural psychology, connecting learning, responses to change and continued professional development to issues of identity and the construction of selves.

Challenging Times

General Practitioners are facing uncertainties with their roles and with the skills and knowledge required to perform satisfactorily. There is growing anxiety about levels of clinical competence as well as accumulating evidence of the poor 'people skills' of many doctors. There have also been a number of widely publicised failures by medics, and in medical procedures, at, for example, the Royal Bristol Children's Hospital and at the Kent and Canterbury Hospital in Canterbury. Moreover, the now infamous Dr Harold Shipman, a Manchester GP, was found guilty of murdering fifteen patients. This appalling breach of trust prompted the Government to announce an independent inquiry into the case, and include the accountability of all GPs. Further, there are accusations that clinical practice is often based rather more on myth and hearsay than sound research evidence (Sackett et al., 1997). Bennett (1998) insists that patients, especially women, need to complain more vociferously about the competence of male GPs: many doctors, she concludes, are ignorant of gynaecological questions, and also insensitive and frequently condescending, and even bullying, towards their female patients. Gendered relations, in fact, at their worst.

Bennett is not alone in her concerns, even if her rhetoric is somewhat strident. Madeleine Reiss (1997) has written, movingly, about the distressing experiences surrounding her husband's death. In informing her of her husband's serious condition the doctor:

> looked as if he would rather be anywhere else, than there with me. He took me out into the corridor, which seemed to be the only place that was quiet enough, and muttered something about the fact that they had found 'tumorous matter' in my husband's brain ... He wasn't unsympathetic exactly, he just seemed uneasy and in a terrible hurry. When he left I felt bewildered and more alone than ever I have felt in my life.

Such experience, she suggests, is not rare. She quotes material from the Royal College of Physicians that many doctors simply do not appreciate the importance of effective communication, while others are disinclined to give it priority because they feel ill-equipped to handle difficult emotional topics, perhaps because they feel threatened by well-informed patients. Reiss raises a series of associated questions, as do other commentators (Morris, 1998), about how doctors are trained; about priorities in the medical curriculum; and, in particular, about the lack of attention given to the emotional/inter-relational aspects of the role, including listening to the patient's voice in the management of illness. These are serious accusations indeed.

Health in the City

I noted, in the first chapter, the Tomlinson Report (1992) and the growing concern about standards of care in the inner-city; and about how the evaluation project into SDL groups, the starting point for the research, was financed from LIZEI monies. And this in turn was a product of the deepening anxiety over standards of care in inner-city areas (as well as of inadequate resources, including for continuing professional development and the support of hard-pressed GPs (Tomlinson, 1992)). The 'inner-city', for present purposes, is used both as a descriptor of actual locations as well as a metaphor, however mixed, for people living in communities pushed to the edge, in an increasingly unequal society. The collapse of traditional sources of employment, growing inequality and material poverty, the decline of traditional working-class solidarities and the emergence of a more fragmented, insecure culture, alongside neo-liberal economics and the Thatcherite assault on public provision and collective responsibility, have, in their varying ways, taken their toll on particular communities, and on the health of many people within them (Hutton, 1995). This is the price paid for what Galbraith once called 'the revenge of the rich on the poor'.

Townsend et al. (1992) have established a clear, consistent class correlation between most diseases, standardised mortality rates and social background. In sixty-five out of seventy-eight categories of disease for men, for instance, standardised mortality rates for social classes IV and V were higher than for either class I or II. Such gradients similarly apply to incidence of heart disease and ulcers, often regarded as the preserve of stressed middle-class, male executives living in the suburbs. Unemployed people, it seems, have the poorest health of all, across a range of indicators (Townsend et al., 1992; Parsons, 1999). A recent report on the health of Londoners (Bardsley et al., 1998), documents the growing levels of ill-health, both mental and physical, in the poorer, inner boroughs of London, compared to middle-class areas. People in the inner-city tend to live shorter as well as unhealthier lives (Benzeval et al., 1995). Social inequalities are alive and kicking.

The Tomlinson Report and other studies (RCGP, 1994) have provided detailed evidence of the above average levels of poor morale, high turnover and emotional stress among the GPs of the inner-city, in comparison to their colleagues in more affluent areas (RCGP 1994). The Royal College of General Practitioners' Report on the Inner-City concluded that urban decay, social division and the crisis of public funding of heath-care services, affect, in a real sense, the health of doctors as well as patients. There is also an ethnic dimension to this, with large numbers of GPs, as well as patients, from minority backgrounds. These GPs are often older, 'single-handers' who may feel themselves at the bottom of a professional pile and increasingly defensive as their practices have come under close and critical scrutiny. Such scrutiny may even, in certain respects, have made matters worse as particular doctors become more defensive and less motivated to reconsider what they do. Others, as will be observed, are fighting back.

Organisational Change

Moreover, this is a period of transition in the management and delivery of general practice and primary care, including, most recently, the establishment of multi-disciplinary primary care groups, designed to deliver local health services (for populations of approximately 100,000). GPs, or at least some of their leaders, have a potentially pivotal role in these developments (Department of Health, 1998). The new system replaces what the 1997 Labour Government considered the inequitable regime of fundholding and non-fund-holding practices. In the former, GPs had direct control over their budgets, rather than local Practitioner Committees. GPs could purchase, for their patients, or so it was alleged, a range of specialist services from hospitals, pref-erentially. Some patients, and doctors, so the argument proceeded, were becoming far more equal than others.

Furthermore, the role of the GP has altered, maybe quite radically, under the impact of various political, economic as well as managerial imperatives. A new contract for GPs was introduced in 1990, placing greater emphasis on a proactive public health duty, on meeting health priority targets in the community as against the more traditional, reactive family doctor function (Launer, 1996). The idea of the GP as the clerk of family records – the trusted holder of a family's histories, in the manner of John Sassall – may be redundant in a more socially mobile and fragmented culture. There is constant pressure on GPs to consider, more systematically, the nature of their work, and to develop clinical practice in the light of the latest scientific evidence and protocols. General practice, it is alleged, can be based as much upon custom as upon sound, scientific evidence. There are also calls for GPs to become more managerial and accountable in prescribing drugs, for instance, as part of the effort to contain Health Service expenditure. And GPs are being encouraged to operate more as team players, working with other profession-als to deliver integrated, and more 'cost effective' and 'efficient' services, in keeping with the current mantras of social provision.

Managerialism

GPs, like other professionals, have become more subject to a range of audits and other managerial interventions, spelling out, often prescriptively, what should be done and how resources are best managed. The highly publicised shortcomings in the performance of particular medics have fuelled this pressure to make the profession accountable. John Holmes (1998) has written that contemporary health services have become a kind of Benthamite world of objectives, measures of outcomes, and protocols. The new right, over three decades, challenged the 'sleepy world of self-serving professionalism' to its core; professionals had 'to render unto Caesar' a more convincing and transparent story of what they were doing and why, as well as how much it cost.

The 'culture' of health service management has changed, radically, over three decades, reflecting the growing domination of public choice theory, alongside neo-liberal economics. Management has to be more proactive and interventionist in the new orthodoxy (Peters and Waterman, 1995; Morris, 1998). Part of this has involved the introduction of more explicit standards and measures of performance, and greater emphasis on output controls, with weight given to results as much as to procedures. But competition and markets were also elements of the new discourse, with contracts, and service-level agreements, as well as compulsory tendering, used to engineer a more competitive, commercial, market ethos in health service management. While doctors might retain considerable autonomy, and new right rhetoric trumpeted deregulation, the times were also becoming increasingly interventionist.

There are other changes running parallel to those mentioned above, including changes to old-style professional demarcations. Professional boundaries are shifting, with senior nurses, for example, taking on roles previously reserved for the doctor, such as performing minor operations and/or acting as gate-keepers to other services. The change may be most conspicuous in the NHS Direct help line where patients telephone to seek advice and direction from an experienced nurse. And the average general practice already has a number of different professionals working alongside the doctor, including counsellors, health visitors, even complementary therapists. Boundaries and roles are, on all sides, shifting, and relationships and responsibilities are in flux.

Such processes can, of course, impact on doctors in different, even contradictory ways. Greater scrutiny of what doctors do, and the application of evidence-based medicine, has led to a number of advances, for example in the identification of high blood pressure, which has meant that malignant hypertension is a thing of the past (Burton, 2000). At another level, fundholding transferred power from Health Authorities in a manner welcomed by many GPs; and some doctors are no doubt exploiting new opportunities provided by primary care groups. But the same or different GPs might struggle with diverse managerial and financial roles, and complain of having less time for patients. Taking over responsibilities from secondary care might also mean a shift in focus towards treating 'illness' and away from a more traditional 'continuity of care' ethic.

The pressure (or opportunity?) has increased in other ways, including educationally. 'Caesar' has insisted that doctors (like all professionals) take greater moral responsibility for their own individual learning in an effort to improve standards. A new discourse of lifelong learning has penetrated the vocabulary of medicine, as it has other professions. Individuals were constructed as autonomous, enterprising learners who should be responsible (for the good of themselves as well as of the wider community) for seeking out education, for updating and for securing their own professional development (Harrison, 1997). We were all, or ought to be, lifelong learners now, but, for doctors as well as others, this begs important questions about the kinds of learning required, and on whose terms; and of the assumptions made about the sorts of knowledge and skills needed, and of what is fundamental and what marginal to the role.

Postmodern Times

Wider cultural change has also affected doctors, including the challenge of 'postmodern' ideas and a new politics of rights and citizenship. There is a decline in deference towards doctors and other professionals and a more litigious attitude to professional relationships: a product, perhaps, of the highly individualistic ideology of Anglo-Saxon societies (Hutton, 1995). There are other postmodern challenges. Ingleby (1998) has charted, over the last two decades, how debates about access to the goods of the Welfare state, with reference to minority ethnic communities, have gathered apace and evolved; as have calls for cultural literacy. The prime concern, in the 1970s and '80s, was whether people were getting sufficient of what was on offer: 'are usage figures adequate?' or 'is the quality sufficient?'. Professionals, it was felt, needed to adapt more to members of local communities rather than vice versa. More recently, there is a shift towards questioning the social construction of illness itself. How is this conceptualised? How do you compose the problem of health and the meaning of dis-ease in the first place? Grave doubts are re-emerging, for example, about illness categories in psychiatry and their Eurocentric underpinnings (Kleinman and Cohen, 1997). Diagnosis is in fact becoming more problematic across all medicine: a client from a minority community may do and think the 'wrong things' but who is right? Basic and contested questions of meaning are raised in this multi-cultural agenda, with no simple recourse to the medical textbook (Ingleby, 1998).

There is a broader, more intellectual 'postmodern' challenge to medicine and the medical model, fuelled by feminism. There are various indicators, which include a growing ambivalence towards scientific forms of medicine and of contradictory, paradoxical feelings about its 'technoculture' (Hodgkin, 1996). There has been a dramatic growth in the use of alternative therapies and of the 'holistic' health movement. Seidler (1994), drawing on feminist critiques, argues that holistic sensitivity brings people into a fuller relationship with the particularities of their own health. Illness becomes more particularistic and individualistic: less exclusively a matter of breakdown in the body, conceived as a mechanical system to be understood, impersonally and universally. In the medical model symptoms are conceived as 'significations' that are universal, forming, in effect, a language of signs irrespective of the person and context. Scientific medicine, so the argument proceeds, has correspondingly disempowered people from understanding themselves and the totality of their condition. Interpreting 'dis-ease', should involve engaging with, and empowering, the whole person in a social and historical context.

Seidler argues that doctors, post-Enlightenment, were given a kind of special scientific authority and that they have, until quite recently, felt secure in this social contract. But this is unravelling at a time when the grand narrative of science itself, and simplistic notions of causality, are under assault (Giddens, 1991). The women's movement, pre-eminently, has reinstated the importance of the particular, the personal and subjective, in the politics of being and healing. The problem for scientific medicine is, as many feminists perceive it, that subjective and emotional life, and more experiential and intuitive ways of knowing, (ironically this might include doctors too), are derided for being unreliable. People, in consequence, can feel stupid about their own health and disparage their own intuitive insights. For feminists the damage is compounded by the historical appropriation of women's well-being by men: scientific medicine is a male preserve which replaced the power that women previously had in the sphere of healing. The history of medicine is, in these terms, deeply gendered. The power of medicine may, in this view, rest on a 'modernist' illusion: that there is 'the truth "out there" which can be known, understood, and controlled by anyone who is rational and competent. The faith that we can accumulate an objective understanding of reality which is true for all times and all places underlies our treatments and our clinical trials' (Hodgkin, 1996). The 'modernist' view, concludes Hodgkin, is under challenge at its core. 'Great swathes of the world increasingly act according to ... a rather different set of assumptions ...' Of course, there are contrary tendencies in the allure of the new gene science and its promises of predictive power; the times, as stated, are paradoxical.

Many medics of course remain sceptical about such observations. Their job, as they might see it, is to get on with the rather more important task of treating illness. A GP academic colleague told me that a severe case of diabetes in a child, in his own child, which was life- threatening, focused the mind wonderfully. If a drug works, abstract questions about causality, and of science, become tangential. There is little sympathy for what might seem over-intellectualised, abstract theorising when faced with distressed and very ill people needing urgent help and treatment. Medicine, especially general practice, is a highly practical profession, getting on with what is required in urgent situations as well as in the long-term care of patients (Burton, 1998; 2000).

And yet medicine is not insulated from cultural change and intellectual challenge. 'Authority' is no longer unquestioned, or science accepted, not the least because the latter produces contradictory evidence, even confusion, and scientists argue among themselves about what evidence actually is, as in the BSE scandal. At one time, Hodgkin suggests, it was obvious what doctors were there to do: to battle against death and disease; and the National Health Service offered a viable means to deliver good care for everyone. Medical research, and its technological by-products, provided the possibility of health for all. But, nowadays, doctors must juggle with many competing ways of seeing the same situation, between themselves and their patients, or between themselves and other professionals. Clinical reality, as perceived by clinicians, has to be reconciled with patients' beliefs, resources have to balance against individual patient need, and ethical dilemmas 'spring "hydra-headed", daily, from medical advance'. As complementary or alternative therapies increase in popularity some doctors embrace them, others remain sceptical. At some point, Hodgkin muses, medicine's modernist, confident 'centre' may splinter into many professional fragments (Hodgkin, 1996).

On Learning

There is a growing debate too about doctors' initial and continued education: its content, adequacy and delivery, and the extent to which they are prepared, or not, for what they do. Many GPs have been trained in conventional medical schools where education was primarily a matter of accumulating a body of discipline-based knowledge, beginning with basic science and moving to more applied forms of medicine. Early clinical training focused on physical rather than psychological diagnosis or on enabling patients to explore and consider their concerns; little or no help would have been offered for improving communication skills. Some institutions have been better than others, but teaching, in general, has tended to be content- and teacher-centred, characterised, too often, by 'ritualised teaching by contempt' (Morris, 1998). Some of this may be changing and the General Medical Council has recognised that there are problems with a factually overloaded curriculum; excessive, lecture-based, didactic teaching; and teaching divorced from clinical context; as well as with an educational culture of rote and surface learning, including forms of assessment which encourage recall without much understanding. The GMC has concluded that the system discourages evaluation, synthesis and problem-solving and engenders a mood of passivity on the part of many medical students. If the emphasis is still predominantly on cognition and knowledge, rather than the emotions and subjective insight, this still represents a changing view from the centre (Dennick and Exley, 1998).

There are, of course, more long-standing critiques, especially of the neglect of the emotional and inter-relational dimensions of medicine in initial training and professional development. The work of Michael Balint and the Balint Movement has a long if marginal history in the profession. Balint drew on psychoanalytic insights and the facilitative potential of the supportive group, in helping doctors manage their anxieties, uncertainties, helplessness and ignorance, which can run riot in some contexts (Main, 1978). As Tom Main has written: '... a doctor, like his patient, inescapably a human being ... beset by feelings and wishes, by subjectivity ... living, experiencing people' who, 'when patients are under strain', experiences some of that in himself. Unless blind defences are in operation, which may close the doctor off from her patient as well as herself. And Simon Sinclair (1997) has chronicled how sociological and critical perspectives, as well as psychological literacy, are often disparaged by consultants as subjective and thus inconsequential.

There is, however, evidence of some challenge to older didactic methods and 'top–down' educational prescriptions, from, among others, the new academic hierarchies of general practice within universities. There is growing interest, for example, in experiential, reflexive, problem-based learning, grounded in practitioner realities. There may be an attempt to seize back some of the initiative for GPs, and to connect lifelong and experiential learning more directly with what GPs actually do, in all its complexity (Burton, 1997). The development of experiential learning for GPs, with its emphasis on patient-centred methods, draws heavily on the literature of adult learning and reflective practice. Stress is placed on examining everyday work and surfacing more intuitive 'theories in use' – taken for granted assumptions and ingrained habits – in a search for insight and greater self-knowledge (Burton, 1997; Pietroni, 1992; Stanley, Al-Shehri and Thomas, 1993). The focus is on experience itself, on thinking of self in interaction, rather than, simply, processing bodies of factual knowledge or responding to a curriculum determined by what others presume general practitioners should know.

It is worth noting that GPs have been participating in continuing education in increasing numbers since 1990, and the introduction of the new contract and a postgraduate education allowance in which every GP principal receives an annual sum as a reward for attending one week of postgraduate study each year, covering topics such as clinical practice, service management and health promotion. This can be treated cynically with the allowance paying for expensive trips abroad, studying primary care in exotic locations (Launer, 1996). But the growth of 'lifelong learning' may also be a positive response to growing professional needs and opportunities at a time of rapid, uncertain change. One problem has been the absence of systematic studies of such learning in action, and of its impact, over time; especially those based on the development of participants' own in-depth reflections on what is done and its effects; and of what might be required for effective and meaningful lifelong learning.

A Gendered Edge?

Medical culture has, historically, been a male preserve. Seidler (1994), among others, has written of the tendency for many male doctors to assume that patients want them to act, for instance, as unquestioned authorities (some do; it is how to respond which is in question). Doctors can feel surprised and threatened if asked too many questions. Some feminist writers suggest that women prefer doctors to be more honest, to admit doubts and uncertainties. But this is an honesty which doctors may have been trained out of as they learn their 'authority' is a burden to bear, in their patients' 'best' interests. Such patriarchal, maybe patronising assumptions are now under challenge (Seidler, 1994).

Feeling a need always to know or to pretend to know, even when in doubt, can be a seductive but deeply damaging illusion. Bennet (1998), from a psychiatrist's perspective, argues that doctors often imbibe the myth of omnipotence in medical training. They may learn that they are being given a kind of sacred knowledge, trust and authority and that part of the contract with society is that they must always be competent; beyond weakness, vulnerability, even doubt. They must learn to cope with their fears quickly, even disguise them. But reality often disappoints, as doctors become tired and disillusioned, not least with themselves, and initial optimism, idealism and commitment are often replaced, by mid-career, with feelings of loss, disillusionment and failure. If omnipotence has to be defended at all costs and inner-discontent and emptiness 'managed', the result is often an endless pursuit of power, drink or new affairs. John Sassall was haunted by the feeling that he ought to know to an extent that the burden became impossible to bear.

The concept of gender I am using here is, of course, partly symbolic as well as being a matter of everyday experience in relationships and work-settings (Connell, 1995). Samuels (1985) and others have argued that gender, unlike a person's sex, is a social construction: a shifting, historically and discursively situated notion, an outcome of on-going cultural inscription and negotiation. The issue, to put it slightly differently, is of investment in identity, and of what can be spoken by men and women in a particular time, place and sub-culture (Whitehead, 1997), and of what has been silenced, or excluded, from the conversation, even within the mind of the individual doctor. Medical culture has been highly patriarchal, individualistic, competitive and blameful, shaping how particular doctors themselves give meaning to their world (McWhinney, 1996). It is a culture that, on the basis of the stories at the heart of this book, is in profound emotional crisis.

Gender, Managing Change and Motivation

Ideas about the place of gender in the cultural psychology of learning, change management, and in response to difficult, disabling experience, derive, in part, from earlier research I undertook into mature students living in communities undergoing major economic and social dislocations. I developed an inter-disciplinary analytical framework – consisting of feminist, feminist psychoanalysis, sociology and cultural theory – to explore how and why particular people chose to enter access to higher education programmes and what it was that enabled them to keep on keeping on towards a degree, often in highly oppressive situations and against overwhelming odds (West, 1996). I wanted to understand how and why certain people, rather than others, were able to negotiate important dislocations in work and/or in intimate life in psychologically integrative ways.

Human motivation, including the capacity to handle change and transcend major life crises, I concluded, had to be understood in dynamic terms. Subjective states are rooted in patterns of relationship and the wider scripts which shape these, over time. Stephen Frosh (1991), drawing on psychoanalytic theory, suggests there are, at the extremes, two potential responses to life crises: a fluid and generative creativity or a pathological defensiveness against change and uncertainty of whatever kind. Frosh argues that the one 'chosen' depends on the strength and cohesion of the self; whether this self is sufficiently secure to cope with perpetual uncertainty and remain open to new experience, or not. We all experience times of fragility: successful progression requires degrees of subjective cohesion and feelings of security. At the heart of the more cohesive self, as well as more effective agency in the world, is an openness to others; to new possibilities as well as to one's own vulnerability and primitive emotional needs for support and sustenance. Continued motivation requires, in short, an emotional literacy, a knowledge of self as well as others, in order to sustain a career, and a life, in times of fracture.

Women, it seemed, in this earlier research, were often better able than men to manage the emotional and biographical processes of transition, in all its dimensions. In the dislocated communities in which I worked, women have often needed, and been better able, to adapt to new roles and demands,

including finding paid work, while continuing to carry prime domestic responsibilities. They have been better at patchworking a life, creating meaning and
purpose from many fragments. This may partly be because women have had
less at stake in the older division of labour and its associated status and
material rewards. They had less to lose in the collapse of traditional sources of
mainly male employment. Many feminist writers suggest that the construction of feminine identity has, in contrast to dominant forms of masculinity,
emphasised co-operation, mutual support, the importance of emotional life
and of sharing experience in all its dimensions. Women, it is argued, have
needed each other, and sharing stories, to cope with multiple, shifting
identities and to keep different parts of a life and self together (West, 1996).

Many men, in contrast, when biographical certainties have shattered, may
be trapped in pretences of coping and a psychological defensiveness, which
can easily collapse altogether over time. Traditionally hegemonic construc-
tions of masculinity have, like the 'male' world of medicine perhaps, involved
the neglect of feelings and alienation from inner emotional life (West, 1996;
Seidler, 1994). There is, at times, a terror of relatedness, intimacy and of vulnerability in male development (Samuels 1993; Sayers, 1995). Men may have
the greatest difficulty in handling the emotional aspects of changing roles and
uncertain times. They can become ultra-defensive in consequence. Samuels
(1993) has catalogued evidence of the defensive mentality among many men
and in elements of the men's movement. Feminism and the democratisation
of the labour market are experienced as threatening and dangerous. Some men
long to restore an older, certain and controlled order, a world where men 'were
like men', and women 'naturally' preoccupied with domestic roles. It is interesting that the men in the motivational research best able to negotiate major
dislocations, were composing more 'feminised' lifestyles, in which more
emphasis was given to intimate and emotional life, to meaningful activity, to
a more integrated lifestyle (West, 1996).

I wanted to know how much such ideas might apply in a culture like
medicine and among GPs, and the extent to which some older, rigid certainties were being challenged at a time of doubt and postmodern fracture at
many levels. Feminism (including feminist psychoanalysis) has destabilised
the sense of confident, ahistorical, coherent, rational, essentialist and unam-
biguously gendered selves. There is, instead, increasing dispute and
uncertainty surrounding what it means to be a man and a woman, how s/he
is constituted and the extent to which gender, as with other aspects of
identity, is open to a variety of different and diverse expressions, even in
medicine. As Andrew Samuels (1993) has written: 'Perhaps for the first time a
category called 'men' can be said to exist ... in the past it has been men who
have defined all the other categories that there might be; men themselves

were simply part of the intellectual furniture. Now, men are looked at in the way in which they have historically looked at everything else.' This book, in effect, takes a long, reflective look at a very 'male' lifeworld, and the health and well-being of those who inhabit it. The diagnosis is that this world can, on occasions, be very unhealthy.

3
Imagining the Good Story:
on Auto/biographical Methods

... There was a novelist in the 1960s called B.S. Johnson who ... was obsessed by the possible truth of a phrase from his childhood; 'Telling stories is telling lies.' This depends on treating 'stories' as a synonym for 'lies'. His mother and my mother would say 'Don't tell me such stories' ... And he really began to believe that fiction was some kind of untruth, unreality ... whereas what you're saying is that these stories are another form of reality, another part of our world – another kind of truth.

A.S. Byatt and Ignes Sodre, *Imagining Characters*

Would you tell me please, which way ought I to go from here?

Lewis Carroll, *Alice's Adventures in Wonderland*

Stories In, and About Research

Interest in the use of biographical, life history and/or narrative research methods – in the stories people tell, why they tell them in the way they do and how they may be shaped by culture and dominant truths, as well as psychological states of being – has developed rapidly in the 'postmodern' moment. Across the social sciences, there is increasing interest in how such methods can illuminate the complex interplay of self and others, psyche and culture, agency and structure, reality and representation, present, past and future, in individual lives and across diverse contexts (Henley, 1997; Mann and Pedler, 1992; Josselson and Lieblich, 1995; Miller and West, 1998; Evans, 1993; Thomson, 1994; Greenhalgh and Hurwitz, 1998). A basic question common to most of these studies has been what enables some individuals, rather than others, to transcend what may be the oppressive clichés of a particular culture or situation, to create more authentic, experientially inclusive, meaningful and empowering narratives and lives. Stories, from such a perspective, are no isolated, individual affairs but reflect and constitute the dialectics of power relations and competing truths within the wider society.

They can also serve as sites of resistance, as a means to challenge dominant regimes of truth. Jerome Bruner (1990) has observed that culture, its myths and scripts, including what it is, or should be human (including being a doctor?), is inside each psyche, as much as 'out there', penetrating deep into intimate relationships and intra-subjective life; shaping what people think and feel about themselves, on the basis of gender, class, ethnicity and sexuality. Telling new stories can, potentially, be a profoundly empowering as well as a subversive act.

The interest in biography and narrative seems, in part, to be a product of transitional, uncertain postmodern times and its associated politics of identity. There has been a movement, over the last two decades and more, to recover the lost or submerged stories of diverse peoples: in particular, in Edward Thompson's compelling words, to rescue the poor and oppressed from the 'enormous condescension of history' (Thomson, 1963). People were possessed of great potential moral and political imaginations and could become agents in the making of their own histories, even in the most constrained and materially impoverished conditions. Inglis (1995) has remarked, in the context of cultural studies, that biography is the way people want to tell stories of themselves at this particular time: as part, perhaps, of a reaction against universal truths which abused many and particular experiences. We are more cautious now about the possibility of final answers, or solutions of whatever kind. Feminism and black and gay consciousness movements have enabled more people to experiment with their stories of who they are, and what they might become, in subtler, more assertive and diverse ways. Identity is seen to be more of a social construct, open to perpetual change and experiment, rather than being fixed, rigid and essential.

Biography, under the impact of feminism, has also switched attention to the small scale and intimate in contrast to the modernist concern with the grand sweep of history. The personal, feminism taught, turned out to be profoundly political too, as the old duality of the social and personal crumbled. Culture – its power relationships and normalising truths – intrudes deep into the heart of every intimate relationship, shaping what men and women think and feel about themselves and each other, and their respective roles. A basic argument of this book, on the basis of the stories GPs tell – when, that is, given space, security and time – is that the concept of latent and/or silenced parts of a narrative applies to them too. There can be regimes of truth at work – about the place of science or the emotions in medicine, as well as issues of power – shaping the stories medics tell. Crucial parts of the story of these 'fortunate' men and women can be marginalised, even silenced completely. More of the silence, and its meanings, needs to be heard and understood.

Narrative and Health Care

Biographical and narrative methods are increasingly used in professional contexts, including, albeit still on the margins, within medicine. A prime focus has been on patients and the importance of story-telling for health and healing. There is, of course, a long-established focus on narrative and its significance within psychotherapy, but there are other areas of health care where narrative methods are being utilised, including in general practice and work with older people (Viney, 1993; Holmes, 1996; Greenhalgh and Hurwitz, 1998). Liz Viney, for example, identifies four crucial roles for stories in the lives of older people. First, stories help people develop and maintain a sense of identity: we know best who we are when we tell stories in which we have active roles; second, stories provide guidance in our lives, preparing for the future and dealing with the past; third, they enable us to impose some narrative order on chaotic events, what Freud termed narrative truth; and, fourth, when others listen to our stories, and value what we say, we can feel empowered. Some of the darkest moments can be at the stage of life when no one listens, or seems interested in what we have to say; when we feel most existentially alone, when others we have known may be dead or otherwise unavailable.

Jeremy Holmes (1996) has written that 'autobiographical competence' – the capacity and confidence to compose one's own story – is central to psychic health. The word 'narrative', he notes, derives from *gnathos* or knowing. Making the unconscious conscious can be reformulated in terms of knowing and owning one's story. Narrative, he suggests, 'turns experience into a story which can be temporal, coherent and has meaning'. It creates, potentially at least, links between past, present and future. Raw material is translated into symbolic form, which allows the sufferer some detachment from what may be painful, even horrific, raw experience. The recognition of the role of narrative in mental health has of course a long history. Freud, as noted, argued the therapeutic power of story and the importance of a narrative truth in 'the talking cure'. If a story makes sense, symbolically, of experience, even if some of the facts are historically elided or distorted, this may still constitute a 'royal' road to meaning and healing. In family therapy, John Launer (1998) has described how some clinicians are moving from the search for normative explanations of a person's problems, towards the new and different story. Selfhood, in this sense, becomes something to be produced rather than discovered, and the story provides a frame for the perpetual, never complete, ontological project of self.

Launer, who is a practising GP, draws attention to the potential role of narrative in various aspects of a GP's work: in taking a medical history; in its counselling dimension, as something that needs to be listened to, allowing patients to create some greater coherence in their histories; and as a therapeutic stance which involves empathic questioning of patients in ways which can facilitate the creation of new meanings and make a real difference to a patient's well-being and sense of agency. Heath (1998) argues that stories between patients and doctors are at the heart of general practice, creating powerful bonds, which can facilitate trust and effective care. But she also notes how stories may be rigid and codified, not the least the stories informing a doctor and her work. They can blind her to a patient's state of body and mind. On average, she notes, the doctor interrupts the patient after only eighteen seconds of the patient's story, closing down some of the possibilities for the story-teller to develop and interpret, in diverse psycho-social ways, more of her/his own narrative, in active alliance with the doctor.

However, such ideas still appear marginal in the medical mainstream. Narrative and biographical methods are certainly marginal in medical research, including research into medical education, continuing professional development or the wider experience of what it means to be a doctor. As Fiona Ross and Liz Meerabeau (1997) have concluded, while there may be many and varied mental maps in health care, and disputes about conflicting scientific paradigms, and between theoretical and clinical approaches, as well as between the specialist and generalist, the most powerful and best resourced, the most normatively potent is a medical model based on the power of 'big science'. The most important facts and evidence are or should be derived from experimental methods, most particularly the randomised control trial. The rest is seen to be largely anecdotal. Even papers at conferences devoted to the education of doctors can be dominated by the lure and status of experimental methods and their language; including control trials to measure the impact and effectiveness of educational interventions in appropriately rigorous and naturalistic ways (as, for example, at the London Association of University Departments of General Practice Annual Conference (AUDGP), 1997). The narrative of big science holds a powerful discursive sway in the hearts and imaginations of many medics. What experimental methods, however, reveal about the complexity of education and people is another matter.

'Big' science means a whole set of procedures in which precise problems are focused upon and 'extraneous' factors removed. Context tends to be stripped away in a language of universal causality and statistical probability. The scientific approach may, over the last decade, have been given renewed life by the emphasis on evidence-based medicine, and clear 'proof' of what works and why, as part of containing costs. The randomised control trial tests the effect of a particular drug, or new treatment, by matching groups for age, social class and gender, in relatively clear and uncluttered ways. An experimental group is given some special treatment and a control group is not, allowing the inference to be drawn, however erroneously, that any difference at the end of a trial period can be attributed, with some probability, to the treatment. Such science, and its assumptions, is often at the core of the stories doctors tell to themselves, most particularly in specialised fields and in public exchanges (Greenhalgh and Hurwitz, 1998).

Greenhalgh (1998) also notes how the medical profession has aspired to an empiricist paradigm for clinical method, and has done so for over a century. Diagnostic decision making, somewhat tenuously, she insists, follows the procedures of scientific enquiry: the discovery of 'facts' about a person's illness is equivalent to the discovery of scientific truths about the wider universe. Under the imperative of scientific rigour, and best evidence, data must be systematically collected: on the precision and accuracy of clinical assessments, laboratory tests as well as the power of prognostic markers, does professional judgement and clinical effectiveness seem to rest. Softer, more narrational and psycho-emotional aspects of a doctor's work – which may be as crucial to well-being as good science – can be squeezed out of the story. 'Knowledge', in the process, becomes separate from the patient, different kinds of knowing from each other, and the science from the doctor's own life history and more tacit understandings. The normalising power of science can, in these terms, disempower a doctor, in the sense that different forms of knowing and insight become disconnected, and a potentially fuller picture is diminished in consequence. Greenhalgh and Hurwitz (1998) suggest there is a relentless substitution of the softer skills of empathy, intuition, language, listening and imagination in favour of a more reductionist science. This, they state, has been the 'most successful part of the modern curriculum' for doctors. It is as if doctors must learn anew matters that may have been known from infancy, but are undermined in their training.

Auto/biography

The term 'auto/biography' requires some explanation, as, by definition, do some of the autobiographical roots of the research. This book, like the doctors' stories, is the outcome of collaborative enquiry, a piecing together of many fragments over nearly four years of in-depth conversations. Sharing time with my collaborators enabled me to understand more fully the autobiographical roots of what I brought to the process and the intertextuality of research. This is another story that often remains hidden.

Auto/biography challenges the normalising fiction of the detached, objective biographer or researcher of others' histories; the idea that a researcher's own history and identity play little or no part in constructing the 'other's' story, or ought not to do, in the name of good, rigorous and objective science (Miller, 1993; Miller and West, 1998). An interview text, to be valid, should be much the same, regardless of who asked the questions. Liz Stanley (1994), talks of an 'intertextuality' at the core of all biography, which has been suppressed in supposedly 'objective' accounts of others' lives. It is as if telling the story of someone else is a purely cerebral, individualistic affair, disconnected from the self and psyche of the enquirer, and their interaction with the 'other', both consciously and unconsciously. The active and contingent presence of the biographer has been excised from the research account, preserving a kind of *de facto* claim for biography and life history research as science: a process producing 'the truth', and nothing but the truth on its subject. 'Conventionally biography enshrines an essentially closed text to which readers have "a take it or leave it" relationship only' (Stanley, 1994).

Michelle Fine (1992) insists that social scientists, most especially psychologists, have persistently refused to interrogate how they create their stories. There is a presumption, as in the natural sciences, that theories and methods neutralise personal and political influences: 'That we are human inventors of some questions and repressors of others, shapers of the very contexts we study, co-participants in our interviews, interpreters of others' stories and narrators of our own, becomes, in some strange way, irrelevant to the texts we publish' as 'research'. She quotes Donna Haraway (1988) who described conventional detachment and distance as 'fetish', a 'God trick ... that mode of seeing that pretends to offer a vision that is from everywhere and nowhere, equally and fully'. Such tricks present fictions of the 'truth' while denying the interests, privilege and power of the researcher. Fine argues, instead, for the reflexive and self-reflexive potential of experience, in which the knower is part of the matrix of what is known, and where the researcher needs to ask her-himself in what way s/he has grown, and shaped the process of research. Such an aspiration assumes no monopoly of knowing but attempts, through collaboration and mutuality, to name more of what is difficult to say or articulate, and to think about its meaning collaboratively. This is a process that strives to bring to the surface power relationships, discomforts, dead ends and uncertainties. Rather than an absence of rigour, or truth, such auto/biographical methods ask much of the researcher, in terms of self-awareness, social and emotional intelligence, sensitivity, integrity, courage and openness. Whole people and whole processes are restored to the text.

Of course, the researcher may still, contrary to what is claimed, impose a story on his or her collaborators. There are power differentials in all research, and this book, in the final resort, is more mine than the doctors', however much it is also the product of collective endeavour. Moreover, empathy, as noted, can be imperialistic too, seducing the 'other' to be unguarded and engaged (Hey, 1999). But if research can engender a process that is open, empathic, imaginative, reflexive as well as empowering – and that is the claim being made – it can provide a means to more profound insights than other methods, including into the process of research itself and its messiness, imprecision and illuminative power. An empowering rapport is always contingent, however, and has to be fought for and maintained over the lifetime of research, as in other human encounters. The story of what really happens when people tell and share stories of an intense and difficult kind, and when they draw on intimate experience, can be a tortuous, fractured as well as, conversely, a profoundly integrative and healing process.

Personal Threads

I suggest that the personality, background, situation as well as the conceptual frame of the researcher always and inevitably shape the way people tell their stories, and how these are interpreted. But if all research is, to an extent, auto-biographical, it can also, through relationship, generate an *inter*-view, a sharing of perspectives, in a living and dynamic exchange. The more the research developed and the more we strove to understand and interpret a life together, the more I shared my experience, and sought to exploit its potential for shared meaning-making. This was partly because I wanted to know more about learning in the context of changes in my own life, and my response to the disturbance of others, as well as of the workings of gender in my life history and relationships. It is important, therefore, to share some of this story, at this stage, as part of setting the scene for the core chapters of the book; except, it should be remembered, the relative coherence of the story was a product of, not a precursor to, the research; in learning about others, I learned far more about myself.

I was, during the time of the research, undergoing major changes in my life and renegotiating aspects of my identity. This included continuing to train as a psychotherapist and negotiating difficult transitions in my role at the university, which led me to question the relative weight given to a public as against a private self. I was beginning to establish more of a 'patchworked' lifestyle, in which psychotherapy and intimate life had greater priority. I was reading the psychoanalytic literatures and seeing training patients. Gender loomed large in this context. Psychoanalytic history and writing are redolent with gendered assumptions. Freud was the good bourgeois, in patriarchal Vienna and reflected his times. He wrote about the enfranchisement of women, for instance, and thought John Stuart Mill's arguments overlooked domestic 'realities'. A woman's role was to keep a household in order, to super-intend and educate the children. He conceded that the day might come when a different educational system would make for new relationships between men and women, but, after all, 'nature' had destined women, 'through beauty, charm, and sweetness' for something else (Gay, 1988). But there was another side to the story in Freud's acknowledgment of the fragile construction of gendered identity (Connell, 1995). Further, as Joseph Schwartz (1999) suggests, the historically very male world of psychotherapy has been shaken to the core by feminist perspectives over the last two decades.

Gender is frequently central to a patient's story in therapy: of, for example, abusive fathers and/or aggressive masculinity and its consequences. What was more uncertain, at least to me, was how concepts of 'gender' related to the actual practice of being a psychotherapist, especially in a more 'masculine' sense. The feminine in the therapist's role seemed clearer, after, that is, so many years of Kleinian object relations, good and bad breasts, psychic nurturing and notions of the therapeutic encounter as a womb. The place and influence of masculinity and fathers, on the other hand, appeared less well articulated, beyond old-style Viennese habits. One view of the 'masculine' tendency in therapy involved a process of looking outwards, helping negotiate wider worlds compared, that is, with a more feminine nurturing and empathic function. But historically, at least, 'masculinity', in a therapeutic context, was often about imposing some patriarchal order and discipline – the word – on a more feminine and elemental being. Patriarchy, Samuels (1993) insists, simply does not like feminine disorder or 'not knowing'. It cannot stand 'moonlike reflection', insisting as it does, that psychotherapy must strive to be a rigorous, empirically validated science. There were clear links here with some of the stories I was hearing from GPs.

Feminist Challenges to the 'Phallus Incarnate'

The feminist challenge, in the writings of Juliet Mitchell (1974) and Janet Sayers (1995), to what was considered an obsessive focus on mothering, and the role of mothers in psychotherapy (as for instance in the work of Klein and Winnicott) made a big impact on me. There had been a neglect of the impact of men's emotional absence and lack of involvement in childcare and domestic labour. Janet Sayers has written of the damage done to everyone – men and women alike – by dominant fictions of masculinity. Most of all a fixation on phallus, power, status and aggression: 'phallus incarnate', as she graphically describes it. This questioning of traditional 'maleness' and a search for balance in their work and life, appears to be important for many male therapists (Samuels, 1993). If, for instance, 'good enough' mothering – a capacity for empathy and relatedness, for 'being with', in Winnicott's language, or to provide sufficient of the good breast experience in Klein's – is at the core of 'good enough' therapy, can men ever be anything other than second best? A therapist friend told me that, for a long time, he felt inferior as a therapist to his female partner who was more 'naturally empathic'. We talked at length about this: acknowledging that we were creatures of our time, place and culture, growing up in the late Forties and Fifties. We both had emotionally withdrawn fathers, who were marginalised in 'caring' roles. And we were both 'raised' to be self-regarding, competitive, striving; men among men in a man's world. It was hard to unlearn some of this, while working to understand what might be important in recomposing our own identities and practice in new ways.

Part of the answer, we mused, lay in our roles as fathers, at least in comparison with our own dads. We had learned to care for and share more actively with our children, however unequal the distribution of labour might remain. We also tended to play the part of pushing the boundaries, encouraging our children to take risks, introducing them to a wider world, alongside caring and empathising. Maybe this was encouraging separation from the maternal embrace. I am tougher in play, more pushy, forceful, competitive than my wife, although she shares some of these characteristics. Might there be some parallels here with the consulting room and the work of a GP?

Was one approach to the question, I mused, to do with the balance between masculinities and femininities within everyone? Might it be, in Jungian terms, about the integration of opposites; a kind of perpetual experiment, a shifting mix of male- and femaleness, according to the demands of the moment; never complete, always contingent? I remain uncertain about this, not the least because, on the basis of the present research, I am more sensitive to the deeply and pervasively gendered inequalities under which most women, including professional women, continue to labour. And I am also aware how much the idea of gender balance is being used by regressive forces in the men's movement to keep women in their place (Connell, 1995). Of course, if notions of 'masculinity' and 'femininity' become detached from specific men or women, and anatomy, they can be reappraised as propensities available to us all. Perhaps, I wrote in my diary, on reading Andrew Samuels, it was partly a tension we all share, between knowledge and emotion, subjectivity and objectivity, informality and formality, law and order, fantasy and language, co-operation and competitiveness. Samuels (1993) suggests that single parents may help us see the lack of nature, as against culture, in the way people can be with their children. Some kind of looser, less rigidly differentiated father and mother function, open to all of us – therapists, GPs and everyone – provided a possible answer.

The Pilot and the Method

The research began, with the pilot evaluation, in 1996. An Associate Adviser in General Practice wanted to discover the impact of SDL groups on working practices, including whether anything changed as a result. This included the quality of communication with patients and colleagues. A checklist of questions was agreed, focusing on the nature and quality of the group experience, on the facilitation, and on each stage of the SDL group's life (to be explained further in the next chapter). There were ten GPs at this early stage, and the Associate Adviser interviewed five of them. All the interviews were fully transcribed, following oral history conventions (West, 1996; Humphries, 1984). The transcript was returned to the GP, along with a tape if requested, to correct or amend as wished. We compared the material generated, each reading the other's transcripts. Some of the findings of this stage of the work are considered in the next chapter.

The pilot, as suggested, begged many more questions than it provided answers and the ten participants agreed to take part in the extended project. I explained, at this stage, that my larger purpose was to undertake a bio-graphical/longitudinal study of health, health-care professionals, and of the meaning of healing and learning in the inner-city. This would focus on how GPs conceived their roles, managed change and the impact of working in the inner-city, as well as the role of learning, and its meaning, in such contexts. I also introduced a time-line to locate individual biographies in a wider historical frame. The information requested (see Appendix) included family of origin; on mother and father, occupations, siblings and so on, schooling/education, professional training, qualifications, significant continuing education experiences, details of medical career (and other careers, where relevant), professional activities including membership of professional bodies, and significant professional/career events.

Next Steps

Of the initial ten GPs two agreed to only two more interviews. And as the research developed, I wanted to broaden the study to encompass more female and ethnic minority doctors, as well as widen the geographical area of the study. From inner-London six more GPs were recruited, via personal and pro-fessional contacts. Eventually nine other volunteers were found, including some from deprived parts of the Medway, an area sharing some characteristics of inner-London, such as large-scale unemployment, poverty, social exclusion and large minority populations. The London doctors were recruited from areas of Haringey, Tower Hamlets, Brent, Newham, Camden Town, Highgate and Islington. Of the original group, six were men, four women and three were single-handers from minority communities. One woman was a single-hander while the remainder were in group practices. Of the second batch of London GPs, four were women and four men. None were single-handers. Of the Medway doctors, two were women and four were men from minority back-grounds and single-handers. The whole sample included doctors with Chinese, Bangladeshi, Kenyan Asian, Malaysian, Sri Lankan, Indian, Pakistani, Welsh, Scottish and English backgrounds. The age range was from late twenties, in the case of one female GP, to sixty-four in the case of a doctor from a minority community. The majority were aged between thirty-five and fifty-five.

Over the four years of the work, there have been up to six biographical interviews, with each doctor, lasting upwards of two hours a time. There were a hundred interviews in the project as a whole. The research, using tapes and transcripts, involved generating themes to be tested and retested, dynamically, in dialogue, over a period. One GP likened the process to 'a kind of extended consultation. I am used to seeing people from time to time and picking up where we left off, continually exploring their stories and what might underlie them, as we're doing in the research.' It was the longitudinal design of the study that brought the process, and relationships, to life, creating, uniquely for many of these doctors, space and time for telling stories. It should be noted, however, that not all of the twenty-five doctors are referred to explicitly in the text. Particular doctors – because of the illuminative power of their story, for instance – figure more prominently than others. All the stories, however, inform the analysis. I have also chosen to make liberal use of direct quotation, partly because of the richness of the material, and partly because such a method takes the reader closer to the doctors concerned, and gives a sense of how they compose their stories.

The Good Story

I have suggested that research is always and inevitably a work of fiction, a representation of experience rather than in some way constituting the experience itself. How then to judge validity, once mathematical criteria are jettisoned? Peter Clough (1996) argues that the peculiar power narrative methods may have is to bring to life experience; and that narratives are best judged by aesthetic standards, including their emotional force, their capacity to engage the reader in the story, as well as the generation of insight and meaning. Conventional measures of good research such as reliability, replicability and verifiability are inadequate to capture the richness and insight of the processes involved. The process has also to be grounded in a moral commitment to truth seeking, even if the idea of a single and universal truth is jettisoned. A.S. Byatt and Ingres Sodre (1995) consider the good story to be analogous, in a way, to the dream, in that this presents experience in vivid images, and offers access to latent meanings and new narrative possibilities. The authenticity and integrity of the material – its validity – become more a matter of aesthetics and verisimilitude (Bruner, 1986), and, as in a dream, the imagination can break free of conventional shackles, for a while, and recover what may have been lost.

Many of the GPs' narratives involved, over time, a process of seeing with fresh eyes, of entering an older story from a new critical as well as emotionally confident and honest perspective. What people have to tell of their experience, motives, and lives more generally, is never complete (Rich, 1972). Individuals may lack confidence, encouragement and/or time to interrogate the ordered and rational claims of professional myths, for instance, in the light of actual lived experience. Furthermore, as Bill Randall (1995) suggests, there is always an unavoidable gap between our selves and our lives: between living and telling, life and life story. Living is always an aesthetic enterprise; an art, a matter of creating shapes from shapelessness. We can make ourselves anew in our own hearts and minds: how we transform things, quoting Hillman, involves the soul taking random images and happenings and making them into more of a whole: the 'novel-ty' of our lives. The good story, and valid research, is a product of making connections across disparate, often disconnected parts of a life, and seeing this with new eyes, and from diverse perspectives and creating more of a whole in the process. Such 'wholes' can speak to others in similar conditions, and may empower them to reenvisage their experience too in more diverse and challenging ways. That, in essence, is the purpose of the study, and the basis of its claim to validity.

On Ethics and Boundaries

A copy of the code of ethics used in the research is included in the appendix. Given the potentially sensitive nature of the material, participants had the absolute right to refuse to answer any questions as well as to withdraw from the research at any stage. I had the responsibility not to push people in directions they did not wish to go, or to assume the role of the therapist. Participants had the right to withdraw retrospectively any consent given and to require that the data, including recordings, be destroyed.

Questions of ethics, most especially those of confidentiality and anonymity, were to become central to the entire project. General Practitioners inhabit a small, enclosed professional world, where many, working in the same area, know most if not all of their colleagues. The problem of people being able to talk openly, and yet securely, was a constant concern never, in certain instances, fully resolved. The boundary between therapy and research was also, on occasions, problematic. Some of the doctors, as will be seen, were stressed and bared their souls, and then worried about what they had said, and what might be done with the material and what would happen to their careers if others found out. Doctors in the same practices worried about what their colleagues might think, and how what had been said about particular people might be interpreted. This, as will be made clear, is a world in which the professional curtain tends to stay closed, at least in regard to particular topics, and even in the company of close colleagues; and sometimes, as will be observed, for good professional reasons.

I reiterated in the final interview, and across the whole study, that anonymity could never be completely guaranteed, and that I would check out with individuals concerned about the use of especially sensitive material. Names and the location of practices were changed, as were other details, as part of the attempt to anonymise. I have gone back to some collaborators a number of times about the use of particular material, and how certain aspects of their identity could best be protected, if that is what they wanted. To link together ethnicity, sexuality, gender and age, for instance, in a particular story, could carry the risk of recognition by colleagues. But where amendments have been made, we have attempted to achieve this in ways that do not lose the essence of the stories, or their narrative power. Moreover, many collaborators stated that they were more than willing to take the risk of being open and explicit, and to keep changes to a minimum, because such stories needed to be told, for the health of the profession, they said. It was their choice, and they had made it.

4
Learning in the City

There are growing concerns for groups who suffer multiple disadvantage and who are increasingly excluded from mainstream participation within their communities. There is evidence of increasing polarisation within London, and a concern for those who suffer multiple disadvantage with regard to health, housing, income, employment and education.

P. Edwards and J. Flatley, *The Capital Divided: Mapping poverty and social exclusion in London*

We can only attend to our patient's feelings and emotions if we know our own, but self-knowledge is neglected in medical education, perhaps because the path to this knowledge is so hard and long.

James McWhinney, 'The Importance of Being Different'

The State of London

'Self-directed learning' groups (SDL) for GPs had their origins in long-standing concern over standards of health, and health care, in inner-London. A recent study of the health of Londoners provides further evidence of the scale of health problems in the inner boroughs, and throughout the whole of London (Bardsley et al., 1998). London is the largest city in the UK, with a population of more than 7 million and is home to the most diverse groups of people in the country, including some of the poorest, as well as the most affluent, sometimes living cheek by jowl in the same area. London, the Report observes, is the most ethnically diverse of all British cities, which can be a major influence in current and future patterns of health (for instance, there are higher rates of coronary heart disease and diabetes among south Asian communities, and so on).

The Report draws together a range of data on Londoners' lives, suggesting some of the potential factors impinging on the health of the poorest people. A third of secondary school pupils in London are, for example, eligible for free meals; the proportion of people living in poverty has increased from 14 per cent in 1983 to 24 per cent in 1992. Nearly 40 per cent of the unemployed had been out of work for more than twelve months, while unemployment among non-whites is twice as high as national averages and among some ethnic groups is over 33 per cent. Two-thirds of asylum seekers and refugees in England and Wales arrive and settle in London. In inner-London one in four women is estimated to have experienced domestic violence. And 40 per cent of the population live in electoral wards that are among the most deprived 10 per cent of all wards in the country.

There are higher levels of acute mental illness too, unplanned pregnancies and substance abuse as well as higher mortality rates, relative to national averages, in inner-London. Brent, Haringey, Newham and Islington have the highest proportions of people living in temporary accommodation: squatters, hostel dwellers, travellers, and those sleeping rough, in comparison to the rest of London and the country. HIV-related deaths were the most common cause of mortality among men aged between fifteen and fifty-four. Inner-London is the focus of the national HIV epidemic and it is estimated that 10,000 adults with HIV infections were living there. The capital also has higher levels of serious mental illness than any other city in the UK (Bardsley et al., 1998). These are the places where many of the twenty-five GPs work and the data indicate, crudely, what life may be like for many patients.

The Health of General Practice

The health of general practice may mirror, as has been suggested, the poor health of many of the peoples who live in inner-city areas. The Black Report (Townsend, Davidson and Whitehead, 1992) noted, over twenty years ago, concern about standards of GP services in some poor areas. The Report referred to the large number of single-handed GPs and claimed that many lived at a considerable distance from the areas where their patients lived, and had little knowledge or interest in the cultures of those areas. They had, the Report alleged, little or no interest in the possibilities of new health centres, group practices or meaningful forms of collaboration with other profession-als. Many were older GPs, some on the point of retirement, and 'there are some who have resorted to work in these areas because they have been unsuc-cessful elsewhere and are exposed here to less criticism'. The Black Report advocated more control over GP appointments, the introduction of an assisted voluntary retirement scheme as well as audits and peer review of standards of care and treatment.

Furthermore, Charles Webster (1998) has written, in detail, about changes in the GP's role over three decades. Some of the old emergencies of lobar pneumonia, empyema and mastoids tended to disappear and GPs were cast, whether they liked it or not, in new roles, responsible for a much wider range of human frailties. Not all GPs, he suggests, were equipped to meet some of these new challenges, including psychosomatic and asymptomatic conditions. He suggests a gulf opened up between 'some of the avant-garde practices' and what he called 'their antediluvian neighbours'. At the avant-garde end of the spectrum, Webster argues, GPs have joined together in group practices to innovate with new therapies, systems of management and research; while at the other end, there is a preponderance of poor services in dismal premises (Webster, 1998). The Turnberg Report (1997) noted that a greater proportion of GPs in London were aged sixty-five and over, and a higher proportion have larger patient list sizes (over 2,500 patients) than in the rest of England. Moreover, the number of GPs in London has fallen by 1 per cent since 1990, while the population has increased, and the number of GPs outside London rose by 6 per cent. Various Health Authorities reported that GP premises often failed to meet acceptable minimum standards. Unsurprisingly, perhaps, morale among some of the inner-London GPs may be especially low (RCGP, 1993). In parts of inner-London, the impetus towards SDL, and towards a quasi-political movement among single-handers, is to be understood against this backcloth.

Self-directed Learning

The London Educational Incentives programme (LIZEI) was established in 1994, and sought to address the historical underdevelopment of primary care in inner-London (NHS Executive, 1998). The aim of LIZEI, as noted above, was to use education, and educational incentives, to recruit, retain and refresh inner-London GPs. A 'fourth R' – reflection – was added so that educational incentives could be integrated into personal and practice development plans, and education could be seen as more of a lifelong process (NHS Executive, 1998). Undoubtedly, these ideas, especially the role and potential of experientially-based, reflective learning, were influenced by the emergence of a new General Practice academic and educational establishment within the Royal College as well as in university departments. The interest in new forms of learning was partly a reaction against the traditional, highly didactic medical curriculum, divorced from some of the realities of the surgery. These ideas drew heavily on the literature of adult learning and reflective practice. Notions of reflective practice, as Ecclestone (1996) has observed, call on the hermeneutic/interpretative sciences in stressing the importance of examining everyday work and surfacing more intuitive 'theories in use' – taken for granted assumptions and ingrained habits – in the search for greater insight and self-knowledge as well as enhanced practice. The focus is on experience, on thinking of self in interaction, rather than, simply, processing bodies of factual knowledge or responding to a curriculum determined by what others presume practitioners should know. A body of theoretical and applied literature has emerged, focusing on experiential learning in general practice and how this, and the professional lives of practitioners, can be enhanced as a result (Pietroni, 1992; Savage, 1991).

The new three-year LIZEI programme was delivered by local Education Boards (which were in fact sub-groups of Health Authorities) consisting of stakeholders, 'working in partnership'. The central budget was £10m for 1995–96; £15m for 1996–97 and £13.2m for 1997–98. There were four elements to the programme: to develop the infrastructure for undergraduate medical education in the community; to pilot variations on existing Vocational Training; to facilitate career development in education and research for LIZEI GPs, and to enable them to devise and implement personal/professional development plans. It was hoped that other professionals might be involved – such as practice nurses and managers, as well as representatives of Health Authorities and University Departments of General Practice – in the design and delivery of the plans. Over 2,000 GPs took part in the scheme, around 85 per cent of those eligible. There is a claim that LIZEI facilitated a major shift in the culture, towards a more reflective general practice as well as strengthening its knowledge base and research capacity. LIZEI also led, so it has been claimed, to a reduction in the isolation of many doctors and boosted their morale (NHS Executive, 1998).

The SDL Project

The particular SDL project that provided the basis for the present research aimed to facilitate learning among groups of general practitioners working in one area. There was a large number of single-handers but also many group practices in a mixed economy of service delivery. The idea was to establish a number of small groups, to appoint a paid facilitator and cover the costs of the Postgraduate Education Allowance (PGEA). Six group practices and five single-handed practitioners were approached by telephone and offered a preliminary meeting to explain the aims and format of SDL. Fourteen general practitioners were recruited, comprising three practice-based groups: one non-fundholding practice (four participants), two fundholding practices (both consisting of three GPs); and a group of four single-handers. 85 per cent of the GPs were members of the Royal College of General Practitioners, mostly working in a group practice. All the single-handed practitioners were members of a local forum for single-handed doctors. Three practice-based tutorials were provided, for each group to consider the meaning of experiential learning, to engage in consultation analysis (participants were asked to keep detailed notes of five consecutive consultations), and to consider critical incidents, such as the sudden death of a patient and/or avoidance behaviour with particular patients. The groups had clear ground rules, including those of confidentiality.

The facilitator led the series of three ninety-minute tutorials involving peer group discussion. Process was seen to be as important as content, and the facilitator worked hard to establish a supportive, secure and confidential space in which it could be possible for participants to share more of their concerns, doubts and vulnerabilities as well as achievements as doctors. The GPs agreed to write a report, as well as keep a reflective diary, and complete a portfolio documenting the impact of the programme, for better or worse, on themselves and their work. They considered specific strategies for change and development and, subsequently, completed a learning plan on future priorities and how these were to be realised (Harrison and West, 1997). The doctors also agreed to undertake preparatory work for each meeting. Time was given to exploring the different management options consultations presented. Each group analysed their avoidance behaviours: those aspects of patient management that GPs may dread and/or refer to colleagues, perhaps because they are disinterested, lack confidence or the cases seem too disturbing to handle.

The facilitator kept detailed notes of each meeting, focusing on the themes that emerged and specific steps participants had agreed to take. After each meeting a report was sent to participants to assist in future planning. They were also asked, shortly after the tutorials were complete, to write a report on the impact and benefits of the project. One year after the final meeting, the ten participants were interviewed and this was the point at which I entered the process.

The Facilitator

Likewise, the facilitator was interviewed a year after the groups finished (a number of the GPs, perhaps significantly, continued to belong to informal SDL groups). The facilitator considered each group to be different, with varied expectations. One group only had a single session and the facilitator felt they became overly defensive, wanting someone with greater professional experience. No one from this group was interviewed. A second group, according to the facilitator, was sceptical towards SDL, emphasising PGEA points rather than any greater expectations. They were felt to be quite a 'closed' practice in which there was a great deal of defensiveness and only limited opportunity for colleagues to meet and talk. Over time, the facilitator felt they came to value the greater camaraderie generated in the SDL sessions. Two GPs from this group were among the ten participants in the longer-term study.

There was a third more 'avant-garde' group, in the facilitator's view, which conceived the programme as an educational opportunity and an extension of a learning culture that already existed in that practice. They were committed to collective and individual development, and to working in the inner-city.

All of the partners were, or had been, participants in a variety of forms of continuing education and professional development, over a long period. There were, in this practice, regular multi-disciplinary meetings to consider problems, including the management of 'heartsink' patients. The facilitator thought the group more honest than most about deficiencies. Three of the group participated in the research.

Finally, there was a group of single-handers who had not previously worked together. They were anxious and avoidant, at first, wanting to deal with practical problems. They were hesitant about exploring more emotional aspects of their work, or difficult professional experience. They were unused to considering difficult patients, and their responses, in such an open way. They were defensive too, in the view of the facilitator, about being single-handers at a time when single-handed practice was under intense challenge. The facilitator thought the group benefited greatly from their time together and progressed well in considering difficult, sensitive material. The group, alongside a number of other initiatives, may have been highly significant in the wider development of a single-handers' self-directed learning movement (Burton, 1997).

Initial Feedback from the Participants

I read the initial evaluation forms and the GPs reported, in the bland way of such responses, that the methods used – such as a needs log – were helpful. The response to the project varied, with the most positive support from the avant-garde practice but also the single-handers. The doctors identified various needs and 'deficiencies' requiring action. There was uncertainty over new clinical procedures, for dealing with dyspepsia, for example; or how to choose among different management options for hypertension in the elderly. All participants identified at least two aspects of patient management they found difficult or avoided, including psychosexual counselling. The doctors blamed their training, and lack of supervision or support in dealing with emotionally complex, including mental health, issues. There were hints in this material of themes that were to dominate the research.

The GPs thought support from colleagues was a crucial factor in enabling them to learn from painful experience, as opposed to becoming defensive and avoidant. Unexpected patient deaths or difficulties with professional colleagues were most often cited as the main causes of severe anxiety and distress. Of the ten doctors, seven devised learning plans, which included attending clinics at local hospitals, working alongside consultants, taking a course on complementary medicine and one on counselling. One GP was doing photography as an antidote to stress and overwork.

The Beginnings of the Research

These first interviews were significant. There were many and tantalising glimpses into the lifeworlds of the doctors: how they managed changing roles and challenging patients, and of the meanings they gave to their work. There was anxiety about committing certain information to tape, and some conversations were more like 'reports' than 'stories' (Polanyi, 1985) – in other words, they were guarded and stiff. I had to gain the doctors' confidence and trust, and the doctors had to see there was something in the process for them. I came to understand, as the research unfolded, the extent to which many GPs have learned, necessarily, to be careful in what they say in the professional world they inhabit.

Yet, if some biographical curtains remained closed, at this stage, there were many glimpses of the personal and professional uncertainties lying behind. These included the pain, for some, in dealing with particular patients and colleagues, as well as doubts about the job; of gendered dilemmas on the part of some female doctors, struggling to balance conflicting demands between a greedy career and a demanding family. There was sadness, too, at lost direction, as well as struggles to reinvigorate careers and to manage depression. There were positive stories too: of particular doctors transcending crises, and of the interplay of personal and professional health in being a happier and more effective GP. Stories, too, of single-handers striving to improve their work and to inspire their colleagues. On occasions the material flowed freely. Some GPs said it was unusual to have someone interested in them, who listened sympathetically.

Knackered

Most of the 'avant-garde' participants were enthusiastic about SDL, one year on. Dr Roy Weber said:

> We were very chuffed indeed and I think we were chuffed for two reasons. One is that we made contact with another local practitioner that we scarcely knew, in fact I don't think I had even ever met the tutor even though we probably work less than a mile from each other ... that says something about the fragmentation of general practice, but I think it also says something about localities like this which are a bit anonymous. We were very chuffed for that reason, we were also chuffed because I think we all shared a sense of frustration with the traditional 'chalk and talk' models of postgraduate education. We had all given up going to the dreary local postgraduate lectures given by consultants who had never been in a GP's surgery in their lives and for us it was a sign of the times that some GP-centred postgradu-

ate education was going to deliver and that we were going to be able to take this into our own hands ... So we were thrilled with it for those reasons ... I know that I took a case that was causing me particular grief at the time. I remember no details of the case whatsoever. I don't even remember who they were. What I do remember was the outcome of my particular case was the typical outcome of these sorts of discussions, of everybody saying 'This is just the sort of messy, muddly, inconclusive kind of work which GPs do. It is the nature of the work, you don't need to feel bad that you haven't packaged it nicely, you don't need to feel bad that there isn't a conclusion that you can present at an academic meeting. That is what general practice is about.' Now that in itself is always very helpful for GPs to be hearing.

Roy drew back the curtain a little:

Yes, I had been in the job for ten or eleven years, full time, which meant nine sessions a week, that is nine surgeries a week, each with maybe twenty patients. I wasn't doing any post-graduate education, either receiving it or giving it. I wasn't doing any research. I didn't have adequate time for reflection. I was doing lots of on-call and I was knackered and at one stage I got ill.

... GPs needed to see themselves as a speciality in their own right and develop their own language, their own epistemology and their own training, post-graduate trainings and my God it has all happened.

Well all the NHS changes, with all their negative aspects, provided opportunities which weren't around before ... 1990 onwards, the contract, the internal market, move towards primary care-led NHS ... a whole variety of things which have dramatically changed the nature of general practice and have created a hell of lot of problems, but have also opened up opportunities. That may also be so condensed that it needs unpacking. Well I think ... all the changes that have taken place can be seen under the umbrella of a move from secondary to primary care and a move from letting general practice get on with its own business in a fairly quiet, low-key way, to seeing that primary care was going to have to be where it was at because it was probably going to be all that a country like this could afford, or a large part of it. And the hospitals may have to close down but the GPs never could. So it was sort of moving the epicentre to general practice and making general practice more visible and more accountable; now this has created horrendous problems in terms of work load for some GPs, but it has also meant, for example, that there was a need to develop people called GP educators, which never existed as a species five years ago ... So it met a need in me, that the culture changed so radically in that five-years period.

He devoted more time to training as a therapist and to educational work:

> And my therapy training has been enormously helpful in that regard because you learn to be a bit more detached and not to feel guilty or responsible for all the craziness and awfulness that is out there; and to find effective ways of saying to people, you know, OK, what are you expecting me to be able to do about it and what did you think you might be able to do yourself and how would these two fit together?
>
> I went off to take therapy and did an introductory course because I thought it was fascinating and very useful. I was very grabbed by therapy personally, not as a client, but just learning about the ideas which made me immensely curious about my own experience and I did some family research which turned out to be personally profoundly important to me in that what I discovered through doing that – I went and interviewed various relatives and I was sort of struck by how that added another dimension to the work that I had done as a client in therapy. When I started my training, if I am honest, I started it at a time when I was getting pretty burnt out as a very, very hard-working, very full-time GP and I thought I might use the training as a parachute to get out. Here was something I could do as part-time training, but could then use to leave the job. But while I was doing it the opposite thing happened. I became very proud of being a GP and felt that GPs were very undervalued in places like this and I also began to think that the whole way that some therapists conceptualise the world was just a tremendously powerful set of tools for using in general practice. So that I became a sort of two-way missionary in a way telling people 'For God's sake appreciate GPs' and telling GPs there is a whole set of ideas and skills which you could use which would make your jobs much more manageable and much more gratifying. So that's the interface that I work at really.
>
> ... I've developed a style of working over the years where I ask myself what can I realistically do in eight or ten minutes rather than trying to solve everybody's lives for them and that style involves a lot of the time handing problems back to people in the nicest possible way and seeing how they might be autonomous rather than taking all the shit on board myself.

Dr Karen Hughes really appreciated SDL:

> Yes, yes. I mean the reason why I agreed to the interview was to support the work because I thought it was valuable, and the effort that the tutor put in. So agreeing to the interview is a measure of support for the project because I thought it was useful. I mean if I hadn't thought it was useful I wouldn't be sitting here, do you know what I mean?
>
> ... Looking back ... I think that the biggest way it was useful is that it actually, all the things I spoke of previously, the strain within general

practice, I think it relieved some of those strains by actually providing a protective time for sharing experiences, because as GPs in a group practice it is actually very difficult to get that time – there is always something else to do. So it was a significant ... where everything else drains the barrel ... it was a significant way of keeping the barrel topped up, if not putting something plus into the barrel, of coping mechanisms. I remember it being useful in terms of ... being very confidential was very important. And people actually talking about things that had happened ... sometimes years ago. And I am talking about something I had discussed, which I don't think I had discussed in ten years, but was obviously still in the back of my mind.

... And I think in just reassuring each other that we were doing okay, you know, that lots of things were happening, but basically the job remained about patient care and about us, and that both aspects were important. Because there isn't really anywhere else that you can do that. You can go and listen to somebody speak and you can often come away with thinking 'Oh God, that's another thing I'm not doing too right!' Whereas this was much more reassuring ... sure it was difficult but ... there's such a thing as a good enough doctor, if you like.

... I deliberately didn't look up any notes or anything, prior to this interview, because I thought well if I have to go back and review, it's not really a day-to-day thing, its an artificial intervention. So I thought it was actually better to rely on ...

... It would actually be more honest, if you like.

... Yes I can, actually. Its just occurring to me that the whole thing has come full circle, in a way, because my self-learning plan, which I did because it was eighteen hours PGEA, otherwise it kept being the last priority, until the very last minute because there was always something that had to be done. But I was involved ... I was interested in complementary therapies at the time, and applied to do a course. Having decided that I did need something completely fresh, almost there was a selfish interest, that it had to be based on what I needed, rather than on what the world needed, if you like ... So it's opened enormous channels.

... I did all of that as part of a self-learning plan. I mean she asked what my educational interest ... was and she said 'Fine. Pursue it, and write it down as your self-learning plan!'

For Karen, the SDL group was one turning point in her narrative:

... one of the things I went away with from the group was that I have to decide what I want to learn. I mean you might say that a learning style is ... one of the most important things about learning is motivation, and I think I went away overall with 'OK, what did I want to learn?'

... As opposed to 'What ought I to learn?' I ought to learn how to ... Oh God there are a million things I ought to learn because they are in fashion, they're the current guidelines, they're the current management strata. I ought to learn what the recent Asthma Steering Group has recommended. I ought to learn that, right? I'm not sure I wanted to learn it, by the time you've been on the third set of guidelines it loses its ... and you realise they're going back to the first set of guidelines and they should have ... Do you know what I mean? You are learning to other people's agendas. And I think what I took away overall was 'What do I want to learn about?' Almost going back to being sixteen and saying, 'What is it that excites me? What learning excites me?'

For Rose Johnson, the group raised questions about practice management:

... I remember I enjoyed the sessions, I remember from the first one feeling that this sounded like a good idea. And especially the critical event one worked very well ... I think that one of the problems this practice has, we have a problem with boundaries, and it is something that is very much a hot issue for all of us as something we are looking at, looking at problems. One of the main, or the main problem that the doctors have identified and have identified for some time, is that the practice has a lot of good ideas, there is good talk, but often we don't actually produce. And there seems to be, there is a real problem with the management side of it, and by the management side of it I don't mean I am necessarily pinpointing anyone in particular, although I think we have, there is a big problem with a member of staff, but actually I think it is to do with these sort of fuzzy boundaries and the way we have set things up, and that is actually something that we're tackling at the moment. We have tackled unsuccessfully in the past and we are just trying yet something else to tackle it, but it feels for the first time it feels that we might be able to break it. But a classic example would, for instance, be that we would end up sabotaging something that could work well by being so egalitarian and all-inclusive that we bring a nurse along and actually take away from the emphasis of what we should be doing by somehow broadening it. And of course it is good to involve the nurse etc., etc. I think that is fascinating because I think, looking back on it, that probably did happen, without identifying it at the time.

Rose was, as she put it, 'hurting' at this time, feeling 'deeply wounded' by a patient's formal complaint. She was considering leaving general practice.

Dr Claire Jones was reconsidering her role and responses, and the tensions between home and work:

Well, I mean people are dumping emotional stress on you all the time in every consultation. I think it is important to try not to absorb it and take it away with you, but it always happens. I think it happens to every GP that you pick up people's emotions and you respond to them like a human being, but I think it's best if you try not to do that and to be an indifferent adviser or observer. But we do get subjected to an awful lot of emotional stress that I find difficult to leave behind at the surgery when I go home and you tend to ... perhaps your family suffers as a result of it ... But I am also very aware that my educational needs I have allowed to become of secondary importance, because of lack of time. And I feel that I really need to read more and to go on more courses, and that's one of our priorities in reorganising our partnership commitments here, and taking on more staff. As soon as we can we are planning to spend more time away from the practice to fulfil our own educational needs.

... Perhaps it is the reflection of the fact that I have a young family, which I didn't have before. But now perhaps I only spend two or three hours a week reading, or attending courses, whereas before I was perhaps spending six or seven hours a week. I mean, I would like to ... to take a week's study leave every two months, ideally. But I don't see that we are in the situation in the practice where we could staff the practice effectively enough to do that.

... It makes me feel inadequate at times, and ... I feel that my patients aren't getting the best out of me. I'm ... I'm aware that, you know, it's a problem that I feel deficient in some areas ...

Dr John Sadler talked about his interest in psychological medicine, but he also felt he had lost direction, for which the project, and its consequences, had provided part compensation but no real cure. He used the SDL group, in fact, to decide to do more writing. John was a Balint-trained doctor, who spent time with patients, using counselling skills and this was what he most valued in the role. But the 'five minute culture', other responsibilities and the growing division of labour, as counsellors were introduced into the practice, complicated his work and feelings. At times, he felt he was left with the coughs and sneezes, and frustration, somatised in an 'excruciatingly painful back'.

The Single-handers, 'Out of the Woodwork'

Dr Ambi, a single-hander, told me:

It was about bringing some notes, going through some episodes in our consultation and discussing through that. And reflecting on what we had learned, where we had made mistakes, and to be open about it in a protected environment, where we were sharing experiences of colleagues in the same predicament, so to speak, and ... she ... ran it with firmness, but she allowed us ... because I ... I think she conducted it extremely well, where she gave us the parameters and set some standards for us to follow to start with: that means no arguments, no ... don't cast any blame on anybody. Those were very nice, very sound.

The most powerful thing is to have ... empathy and humility. Those are the two things we need ... to be successful with colleagues. Obviously we have to learn to accumulate knowledge, but without those two you can't get others to work with you and are not effective at all.

Yes. The problem with anywhere is ... if anything is issue-based rather than personalities, then we can solve them ... any solution. So even in the self-directed learning group there are personalities: they will start trying to dominate, 'Do this, do that!', so one has to tell colleagues 'That's not the way to do it, let's look at the issues. You have a point of view, let's write it. You have a point of view, let's write that.' 'I have a point of view, I totally disagree with anything you all have said.' That doesn't matter. Does it solve the problem? That's what we must look at ... I realised that the single-doctor practices have been undermined, and wherever you went people were feeling on the one hand they were very very sorry, and on the other hand they were undermining us saying 'they are no good'.

... Even our colleagues who were involved in LMC and ... big practices and all. They were feeling very sorry for GPs in single-handed practices. In a way rightly, on the other hand they were feeling sorry because we are no good and we have to be given a helping hand. But that was not my perception of it. I felt that we are stronger, we can manage, but we need peer support. So I spoke to some of my colleagues and we started this and it went from strength to strength ... I think the tutor also had the same idea. So it clicked. It clicked.

The thing is what we did was outreach, we went out and spoke to GPs. I had some experience, so to speak, a bit of outreach because I interacted with a lot of my single-handed GPs. I was the facilitator for that.

And we had outreach activities like practice-based meetings where I went along and got people going, talking about ... the deprived, the isolated type of GPs ... So I knew where the problem was because most of them didn't have time to go anywhere. So they wanted problem-solving educational activity.

Dr Apoorv explained a critical incident he took to the group:

... I had seen the person the night before. There wasn't anything ... I think I diagnosed something like pyelonephritis. And another general practitioner had seen him and did a test which came as positive for proteins in the urine, so that sort of indicated he had a prostate problem. But subsequently the backache was due to a leaking aneurism and he died two days later. Things like that, I mean we all carry this guilt. It's as though we ... had I thought of this, maybe I should have admitted him to hospital ... Those sorts of issues all came out and one could ... I wouldn't say rest assured but feel there are other people with similar experiences ... It's not as if 'Oh that's a great mistake', but it gave certain comfort in believing that ...

... Because I had the singular instance of an aneurism, yes. This particular aneurism, yes I discussed with the group because another GP had the similar situation where somebody dropped dead two days later. So it was like a common problem ... I think I just keep reflecting over and over again, talking with people ... and when one dreams, you know, various things, like that I think somewhere I find these things can make some connections ... As opposed to shutting yourself off from other people's emotions.

Dr Ambi had shared a difficult management problem:

Yes. In fact I had a very difficult situation. There was a lady who I subsequently found out was trained as a nurse, who had moved from an adjoining practice to this practice and this did really wake me up in the middle of the night and I had to think ... She came with a history of saying that she had a brain tumour and she'd been in this group practice and she goes from one doctor to the other. Nobody seems to be managing her very well. She's under a drug, also, she named the drugs, and 'Could I join your practice?' ... I've got a very open policy ... at the moment the door's open. And if it's open it's open for everybody, and if it's shut it's shut for everybody. That's the sort of policy I make, I don't discriminate even if it maybe is a difficult personality. And she rang me and wanted to join us and I said 'Fine, if that's what you feel.' Anyone can join the practice as far as I'm concerned. And she did join and then the first thing she came out with was 'Can I have ten vials?' She's got this bad brain tumour and migraines. A very plausible lady. And I said 'Look, I'm not very happy with this, but certainly until I get more information I will give you a limited supply.'

... And then she sort of regularly called in the night for drugs, she was saying she had such bad headaches and various things. And she would be on something like eighty-four vials for a week from the previous practice, so I had a great job of trying to cut it down. And then there was this husband who comes on and says she's in trouble she's ... the whole family was completely dissolving ... dysfunctional. And in the end I managed to get her off the drug, and subsequently I decided this is an addict although she was under the guise of having migraines. It's a very complicated case. And during that time, I must confess, she did manipulate a lot and have great difficulty getting herself off the medication, and that led to ... I do remember one instance where I was looking after the children as my wife had gone to a conference somewhere, and suddenly the Practice Manager rang me at home. During the time I was looking after the children there was a locum here. She rang and said, 'Sorry to disturb you at home, but the situation is that this lady has come with a photocopy of a prescription issued by a deputising doctor and she wanted some more drugs.' I said 'No!' and the locum was told not to issue any more. But then she comes with these plausible stories and everybody gets drawn in and it's very difficult. And I had to tell her that and immediately my anxiety levels went right up, roof high. And then I put the phone down and I think in the meantime the children had done some funny thing somewhere, I think spilling somebody's dinner, or something like that, and I just screamed at them, and completely frightened them. And I couldn't understand myself why I did that. But it was a situation where it had got to me ... the barriers had broken down, so to speak, and it really upset me ... This is regarding how to shut myself off, I find occasionally I have problems.

Ambi said the group helped him, but the experience continued to bother him, and he was sometimes haunted by a sense of inadequacy. He was not alone.

Wider Evidence

SDL groups, such as these, have been subject to many evaluations, as have LIZEI projects as a whole (NHS Executive, 1998). SDL was considered useful educationally, and also in networking and identifying resources above and beyond particular practices. The groups, it was claimed, enabled GPs to deal more confidently with non-medical issues such as partnership splits. Mental health issues had been given more priority, with problems such as bereavement counselling, substance misuse and patients with 'multiple problems' being dealt with in the groups. Carmi and Hiew (1997) have claimed that SDL involved a silent revolution, transforming some of the lives of a lost regiment of GPs. The key was the fact that the GPs owned the agenda, and in a context of wave after wave of official initiatives on medical audit, health targets and evidence-based medicine, as well as new discoveries and technological advances, constantly hitting practices. Some people kept their heads down, but the SDL groups offered a space where they could begin to shape the agenda. 'The significance of collectives of burnt-out doctors in mid-life crisis, getting their act together to update themselves to survive in their jobs, would have been lost in this era of widespread social maladjustment and skills mismatch, were it not for the strengths demonstrated by SDL group members ...'

Strong claims, and the initial narratives of the ten GPs highlighted the many positive effects of SDL. These included better planning of education and the importance of peers to effective learning. The groups offered some space to raise tricky issues in confidence. Moreover, the first interviews identified certain themes that were to form the substance of the whole study, including how many of the doctors felt outsiders in a male, rigid and, at times, racist world; on the psychological distress of some GPs, and how difficult, even dangerous, it can be to talk, and about the influence of gender in everyday encounters and assumptions. Before exploring these themes in particular narratives, I want to tell a story about the uncertainties of auto/biographical research, in the unpredictability of general practice.

5

A Wet Monday in June

... we in our society do not know how to acknowledge, to measure the contribution of an ordinary working doctor. By measure I do not mean *calculate* according to a fixed scale, but, rather, *take the measure of* [original emphases]. It is not a question of comparing the doctor with the artist or with the airline pilot or with the lawyer or with the political stooge ... It is a very different matter when we imaginatively try to take the measure of a man doing no more and no less than easing – and occasionally saving – the lives of a few thousand of our contemporaries. Naturally we count it, in principle a good thing. But fully to take the measure of it, we have to come to some conclusion about the values of these lives to us now.

John Berger and Jean Mohr, *A Fortunate Man*

Of Courts, and Complaints

Conventional stories of doing research, like accounts of medicine and the doctor's role, often suggest a predictable, ordered and linear process from which much of the chaos, confusion and doubt that can beset the researcher, and research, has been exorcised. Research, however, in the unpredictable setting of a doctor's surgery, and in working biographically, can be a messier matter. Anxiety, and a hint of chaos, may be part of the lived experience of the researcher as well as the doctor while boundaries – between research and therapy, for instance – can become confused in the face of specific distress.

And this happened on a wet Monday in 1998, on arriving for a third cycle of interviews, eighteen months into the project. I was well prepared that day, or so I thought. I had read the previous transcripts, listened to the tapes more than once, including on the drive to London. I made detailed notes on the content and process of the previous interviews and generated some themes I hoped we might explore together. I was scheduled to interview two doctors, either side of lunch. The process would begin, as I imagined, as interviews tended to, by sharing our responses to the last transcript. Relationships with the two doctors, by this stage, were well established and fairly positive. The day was mapped out, with clear objectives.

June was a wet month, one of the wettest on record. The journey to London was fraught with traffic jams and I was anxious about arriving late. Doctors were busy people and I worried that I might waste precious time. I worried too about losing people's goodwill in the study and that particular individuals might withdraw. I arrived, as it turned out, early for the interview with Sarah Cotton, as the traffic eased and the rain stopped. But she was very late, and clearly agitated on arrival. She apologised, profusely, for keeping me waiting, made some coffee, which we took to her room. She was clearly upset and distracted.

Plans were quickly abandoned as she took out a piece of paper from her handbag and slapped it down in front of me, on her desk. 'You want to know what it is like to be a GP, Linden, here's your answer', she said. 'Shall I switch on the recorder? I asked. 'Yes'. A patient had taken her and the practice to court. The patient had arranged for his mother, who was also a patient within the practice, to see a specialist, privately, and had sent the bill to Sarah. He was annoyed with Sarah for not being there on the day when he wanted his mother to see her. Sarah refused to pay the bill because, she felt, it wasn't her practice's responsibility. But it led to an argument and time spent in a Magistrates' Court. Sarah was forced to spend precious hours preparing the case, writing statements as well as being interviewed by her solicitor. It was intensely unpleasant, and turned out to be unnecessary because the judge threw out the case in the first ten minutes. There was no specific contract, he declared, between an individual practitioner and a patient, at least in this case, not the least because her partner had been available, that day, to see the mother. There was no reason for Sarah to have to defend herself at all, the judge pronounced. But the patient was still not deterred and was now taking her colleague, and her behaviour, to the GMC. She had seen the patient's mother, but had refused to do a home visit shortly afterwards. Sarah had to take a morning off work for ten minutes in court and was forced to employ a locum, at a time of financial difficulty for the practice. Such patients demanded time and attention, like demanding children, even when she was on sick leave. The man was abusive to receptionists. Doctors, Sarah said, were supposed to be there, never ill, open all hours. She was very angry.

Expectations

Sarah filled in more detail:

> Yes that's right. In a nutshell he felt that we were not able to give him the service that he wanted at that particular point in time, which was a home visit from myself on a day when I had to go to visit some other emergencies and my partner visited them the following day. I was away on sick leave

that day and so my partner visited and failed to make a diagnosis of something that is intermittent anyway and wasn't particularly serious. And when he called for a request for a repeat visit, my partner said he would go and because he didn't want my partner to go to visit his mother, he decided to take his mother elsewhere, even though they could have had an appointment to see me the following day, or a couple of days later. And so he felt that the service that he wanted at that particular point in time, from an individual, was not available to him, so he felt that we should be responsible to pick up any bills that he had incurred ... Producing statements, being interviewed by solicitors, communications and correspondence with defence unions and so on and so forth. Really it was a first for the MDU [Medical Defence Union] as well, because the claim was only for £120, £110 for the consultation and £10 administration fee, but they said that we shouldn't pay it. They felt very strongly that we shouldn't pay it. It was the first time they had ever had to deal with such a claim. Because it wasn't really a matter of money because they would have settled for less, but they felt that it would be admitting in a way liability because at a later stage he was bound to go on and address a formal complaint to the Health Authority for failure to diagnose that particular condition during the home visit that occurred. And then the complaints committee would say well if the doctors were not in breach of their contract, why did they pay this bill.

She asked if I wanted to know about a second case, while we were at it, from the previous weekend. She had removed a patient from the practice list for aggressive and abusive behaviour. He had complained to the practice, and to the General Medical Council, that Sarah was unfit to be a doctor:

Right? This is a particularly obnoxious family. They were so obnoxious that they accused our senior receptionist of racial discrimination and she is coloured! Yes, yes. And the General Medical Council sent me this by Recorded Delivery at the weekend and I think that it is unreasonable, it is unreasonable but I am going to write back to them, put it on file, that I felt that the behaviour of this family was really unreasonable, so that it is on record, because they do say in their letter that although they have decided not to take any action at all, we are under no obligation to comment, that they do keep this confidential matter on record and if we have any further complaints regarding the practice within the next two years, then that is taken into consideration.

Sarah pushed two more letters in front of me. I never opened my research file. The family complained about being removed from the list and she had written to them to say the relationship had broken down, and it was best to register with another doctor. Alternative doctors and practices were suggested. Sarah thought a great deal about what would be best for the patients. She smiled, however, for the first time, at the thought of passing the family on to another GP. She had talked with the man the week before, saying the practice staff no longer wanted to deal with him and his family because their behaviour was abusive. But the whole family threatened suicide if she abandoned them. They were unstable and the eldest daughter had committed suicide:

> so I agreed to take them back on my list on the proviso that they would not abuse the system that we have. But they abuse the system constantly with every member of our staff. They were involved with arguments with all of the reception staff. They insisted on appointments at times when no appointments were available and they would perhaps not turn up for the appointment ... They would take emergency appointments with them, the nurse, for example, for complaints that were really quite routine and make the nurse run late when nurses are not supposed to provide emergency appointments. They have fixed scheduled appointments. And so I had all my staff complaining about this family, all of my staff saying to me, can you please remove this family from your list because we don't want to deal with them any longer. And that's really just naming some minor aspects of their behaviour because to go into it in more detail, on a personal level, they were not taking the advice of their doctors either when it came to treating their medical conditions, but we were prepared to continue to put up with them as heartsink patients but our staff were complaining bitterly about having to deal with these people.

There were particular twists to the tale. This family wanted to be on her list partly because of Sarah's ethnic background, which was the same as theirs. They were strangers in the city, and felt in an alien culture and she would understand them. They would not go to any other surgery, with doctors whom they felt would be unsympathetic. The family had a strong father figure at its head – something of the tyrannical patriarch, as Sarah put it – and he found it hard to take advice from a female doctor. He had preconceived ideas on everything, including his own health and was convinced he was always right. Yet if he was ill it was Sarah's fault, for removing him from the list or for being unavailable.

Sarah described her feelings when such 'heartsink' patients walked into her surgery, where the interview was being held:

> I think you brace yourself for the onslaught before they come in and allow yourself a little bit extra time and try to be more patient. But it is awfully

hard to manage somebody who you know is not going to take any notice of whatever you are going to say to them.

... I think there is some underlying anger yes, that they feel that they are perhaps not getting what they want and that makes them angry and you know that whatever you say to them they are probably not going to take the medication, or take your advice, so it sort of deters you initially from making too much of an effort to do that. So I think it is just very disheartening having to deal with people who you know are not going to take your advice and they've got their own fixed preconceived ideas of what is good for them. They would rather listen to their neighbours and other people that they know rather than their own doctor. It's frustrating. But I am very patient. I was very patient with this family, extremely so, they were on my list for five years. And now I have this scenario where I am bumping into them regularly and you know we have been through all this unpleasantness and we can't get away from it. It is a constant stress.

No Getting Away

Maintaining boundaries was difficult for Sarah, on her own admission. She could not escape the problem, even at the local church. She tried to ignore the family but was frightened her name might be sullied. Wounding comments were spread around by unreasonable people, and might be listened to by other patients. A priest became involved and told her, "'Look Sarah, this family, they have got a name for being difficult to deal with. He has got a brother and his brother and his family are also equally difficult to deal with, to a point where they have got a name for it." And so he said "just try and ignore it."' But it was hard. Sarah returned to the court case, amid feelings of being appalled and angry about having her time wasted. The family warned her that they would not rest until the matter was resolved, to their satisfaction, and she agreed to take them back. She asked if they really wanted to be on her list when she didn't want them. But they would not take no for an answer and now they had complained about her partner. The complaint, in going to the GMC, would be on record, even if dismissed. It was a slur on her professional reputation, and the practice, which annoyed her.

Managing Emotions and Partners

We talked about managing emotional distress and confusion. She tried to talk with her GP partner, the practice manager and her own husband. But it was hard to take matters home and there were the children to worry about. They needed to come first, because her young son was unwell and seeing a specialist. She also felt that her GP partner had been unreasonable, leaving her in the lurch for three days, at short notice, when she, Sarah, had been ill and there was a flu epidemic:

> ... 'How do you want to deal with it?' and she said 'compassionate leave' and I said, 'Well there is no provision in our contract for compassionate leave at short notice, so you really have to take it either as annual leave, or as extra days' leave which, if there were a locum employed, you should be responsible for that locum. So I think it is important to talk about problems that are bothering you and to get them out in the air and to deal with them, because if you bottle them up, then I think it makes for a worse situation when the next problem arises because you have already got problems that are bottled up.' So we discussed it and I am a little uneasy about the same sort of thing happening again and I sort of worried that perhaps my partner is becoming unreliable, but I think I have expressed the fact that I was not very happy about one or two things to her in a personal meeting, partners' meeting and I think that is the way you have to deal with problems in a partnership, you have to try and deal with them as they occur and to discuss them and to decide how they should be managed best.

Matters were far from resolved, and there were tensions at home too. Sarah had been in a previous practice partnership that dissolved. You needed people to rely on in time of pressure, and sometimes they were hard to find. After a pause, I mentioned a recent study of thirty GPs and their responses to complaints. Feelings of shock were followed by anger, depression and even the contemplation of suicide on the part of some doctors (Jain and Ogden, 1999). Many of the GPs claimed to have learned from the experience, but some also said they were practising more defensively and others had tried to switch themselves off, emotionally, from their work, avoiding risks, if at all possible. Sarah was unable to switch off.

East Enders

Dr Ambi is a single-handed practitioner who works in the East End. He dreaded Monday mornings. There was always a big queue waiting to see him. Ambi felt obliged to see everyone first thing on Monday morning. Many patients, after all, were from backgrounds like his, and he knew them personally and their experiences. There had been a difficulty the day I arrived and Ambi was feeling upset and bothered:

> ... there is one patient who came in to be seen early in the morning, so I came at 7.30 to see the patient first and then I thought I had sorted her out

and gave her a prescription, did this and that, and arranged for her to be seen by a specialist.

... She had a severe headache and a pained face and congested nose. She had been seen by an assistant on Friday. The patient was not satisfied with the outcome of that and she is a health worker, she is not happy carrying on like this, so what about an immediate consultation with the specialist. In fairness to her she wanted to see that specialist even privately, so I rang the hospital to arrange a private consultation and the consultant was not available, even to see her privately, because he has gone on holiday. Then the mother comes into the scene and she wants her sent to the specialist now. It is not just the patient, this is not easy, so you have to adjust to all these different demands. So the patient feels that she has pressurised me, but the mother feels that her daughter is not getting better and I should do something about it. And in the middle of another consultation this call comes through from the daughter saying that the mother is insisting and all this.

Ambi was busy with another patient, and wearing gloves:

... And you cannot write, she [the mother] gives a number, you must ring this number now, I have spoken to the hospital and you cannot write with gloves on. So I write with the left hand and I get annoyed, so I keep telling her, 'Look here, I am in the middle of a consultation, you may not realise that.' They are intruding on somebody else's time and however you put up with that and somehow write it down and then the next question is – 'How soon can you arrange it? I want this done now.' So I said 'give me an hour to sort this out and then come back to you. I will somehow arrange something for her.' Not that it is a life-threatening situation, but for them it is such an urgent business. And this is general practice where every individual comes with pain or acute condition needing immediate inter- vention, or it is a sub-acute condition where they can wait and allow us to deal with other problems and get back ... You see it is impossible ... And the GP who has to pick up the pieces, keep on chasing, chasing. So if it is a medical thing which I am not able to meet I can understand. The high expectation is the most difficult to meet. So it tells on you. So that puts – you can't deal with the next patient with the same amount of vigour and attention because your mind is, I am sure in psychology you would understand, my mind is so engrossed that the next patient doesn't get the attention and care himself.

Ambi explained how, in these confused circumstances, he could give a wrong prescription:

Yes. On the other hand the expectation is so high and patients are so anxious ... we have to face the music whether it is NHS or a private referral, we have to somehow – a lot of people think it is only NHS referrals, we do private referrals as well. That is even more demanding than NHS referrals because 'I am prepared to pay, Can you arrange it now?' And you ring one place, another place, and in time I give up, and I say, 'You ring everybody and come back to me and I will refer you.' Then they come back and they want a letter today, now, tomorrow.

The first patient and her boyfriend, and later the mother, came to see him, again, later in the morning; the insistent and impatient mother pressuring the daughter to act, and an uncertain boyfriend who dithered, plus the daughter caught in the middle.

Ambi was worried, too, that morning about money. He had a better than average workload because of where he worked but money was scarce and he had staff salaries to pay as well as the hire of the premises. He was ambivalent, at such times, about being an independent contractor. While it gave him independence, there were disadvantages too. Like having to manage the surgery, pay the staff, and create a learning organisation. There was something else that morning:

> I had my manager, he is a very good manager, but he said that he can't, his pay is not high enough compared to the neighbouring practice, which is a lively practice, not big, about 1,000 patients more and he said that manager rings him all the time and I said 'Well, that is credit to you. That doesn't mean that you should get higher pay than him.' He gets higher pay than him despite looking after a bigger practice. So I feel bad about it, because I am a conscientious person in the sense that I don't want him to feel like that. If he feels like that then there is resentment. So I clearly told him – 'Look here, I don't want you to feel unhappy about it, but I want to put the cards on the table, see the rationale of my argument.' He agreed, but then that again is a burden on the person who is running the show.

And there was me to deal with too. Ambi laughed saying he hadn't read the transcript, Linden, '*so there*'. We laughed together.

Committed to Staff, and the Practice

A new document on multi-professional education had arrived on his desk. He was committed to education because it was important to show how small, single-handed practices could be developmental. It was his mission in life:

CPD [continuing professional development] is what is necessary for all of us and I am trying to bring them something, to devise some instruments, develop that in this surgery, on my own, with my staff collectively. And to show it as an example as to how in small practices this can be done. If my staff are not happy at the rate of pay they are getting they are not going to be forthcoming with my high expectations. So I have to struggle with this situation. Because I want to bring this surgery to a standard where this can be seen as an example for others and, as you know, I am interested in multi-professional education. So one of my feelings why people don't listen to teachers, or tutors, is that there is a lot of hypocrisy in the teachers who go round and teach others. You go to some tutors who have come to me before. You go and see them in their tutor surgeries. Things are not right. If you question them succinctly you will find that everything is upside down there. But they come to teach us. I don't want to be in that position. I want to show it by example and so I am struggling with all this and I have a family to look after, I have to earn a living, have to get the system right, want to teach everything. But maybe I am trying to do too much. I am not sure. But that is something that I like to do and in the middle of this, this dissatis-faction, what happens in life is people forget from where they came. Members of my staff, all of them are still with me, never left me, because I always tell them – 'Look here, let us grow together. We have to learn, we have to adapt, we have to change, but whatever may be the fruits of our labour, we will share it evenly, but don't expect miracles from here.' And this is the gospel I have been telling everybody and I think they are a very happy bunch here. But sometimes external influences and others talking about these things and it has an effect on them and they come and say this and it is upsetting to me.

He wanted to deliver the best service as a single-hander from a minority community. He was hurt by constant criticism. He set himself a hard and demanding agenda and the more he involved himself in GP education, the guiltier he felt about neglecting the practice:

> ... That is why I feel guilty about it. You can see I have given priority to other things and then left this to fester or whatever. It is not that – I am not a poor paymaster, but my expectations are very high because I want everybody to do audit and I want everyone to come and tell me what is wrong with me.
> ... Yes, yes. That I am demanding too much from them. But what convinced the health authority to give the increase that I wanted, in spite of all this squeeze they are under, is because I convinced them I am getting a lot of work done here in order to set an example to other surgeries.

Ambi was a man of many ideas. All the staff had agreed to produce learning portfolios. He designed audit and encounter forms in collaboration with them. He was constantly telling the staff to speak openly if there was anything wrong:

Because I am open to criticism. I am quite happy to accept all that they say about me. I expect others to be like that and it is not easy for others with me. But I don't take revenge. I don't take revenge. I don't blame them for failing. I don't. Because I look at this place as a learning organisation. So I get irritated when others don't look at it that way.

Work Pressures

Yet Ambi was well aware of discontent about the pressure of work. The reception staff had analysed twenty sets of relevant patients' notes to measure how many women patients, from the relevant age cohorts, had been given family planning advice. The staff resented the time but Ambi stressed the benefits of the 'learning practice':

... And there is another instrument I am thinking of to have a practice activity analysis. How the practice is working ... You get – a receptionist for example to do a bit of activity analysis. She does it herself and then I go and tell another practice that this is what I have done. Instead of me going and telling them, you get the receptionist also to go and tell them. See what we did, I did, I did. And if she can be empowered to do that then she feels very good and she has potential to go up as well.

... We refer patients to hospital and the hospitals send back letters saying that we have not received this letter. Now if we can analyse how many letters are sent out, how many have reached them, because we personally send the letters and we have a courier who takes the letters. To make sure these letters reach them we send them by courier. Sometimes it is posted, sometimes. So all this has to be analysed. It may not be a big job, it is a simple thing to do. But in the process what we are doing is we are keeping an eye on how hospitals are responding. So how I see it is if a simple procedure like this can be done by a receptionist I don't have to do this. The receptionist can do it easily and if she puts it in her record and then passes it on to the hospital saying that this is what we did, it will definitely bring about change in them because moaning and moaning doesn't make any change.

... So if you get the organisation right and empower one of my receptionists to make sure that these patients are monitored for folic acid, then they are contributing to my clinical outcome. And so this is what I am talking about. I think if we develop that then when they talk about multi-professional learning and – one thing I don't believe in is this clinical demarcation between clinical responsibility and non-clinical responsibility. There is a big grey area in between where we are all contributing to the clinical and non-clinical outcomes. And that is where efficiency can be brought in and effectiveness can be brought it. Am I right in thinking that way? So in order to do that we must make them feel that they are also contributing to the clinical outcomes. Why not? What is the problem with that? Just because I am a doctor or a nurse ... they must be able to challenge me. This dynamic is what I am trying to develop here.

Emptiness?

I asked Ambi how he took care of himself. He said that was another story:

> ... I want to tell you about what happened over the weekend ... I am so engrossed in my work and my mind is working overtime all the time, even when I am at home... and my eldest daughter said to me – 'Daddy you are going to lose me soon, because you don't sit and talk to me' and she had a go at me and my wife as well and so this emptiness is something which I may not have picked up. And she said – 'You don't spend time with us, you don't sit and talk' ... My children are nice children, they don't go out. They stay at home and do all sorts of things and we have these orthodox strict regimes and all that. They put up with all that in this country. But at the same time we think we are giving the best for them. We try to do everything. But when she came out with this ... I have two other daughters. So all this stemmed from my last girl. She is doing her GCSEs now and she came and cried the other day because she had missed a question. She was aiming for A and she is not going to get it. And she can't get in. She wants to get into medicine. So I am struggling with what I should do. Should I do all this and then be a proud professional or am I leaving an empty space for my children? It is something which dawned on us yesterday, no on Saturday night actually, only we had this bust-up. It is a bust-up, the children weren't giving, they said nothing doing, whatever you miss you are not doing enough as far as the emotional aspect is concerned. Physical and financial aspects they recognise that we do all what we can, but emotionally not doing at all. So I sat and listened and I thought to myself – yes I think you have a point, my eldest daughter, and believe me the next morning, I rise and am very happy and our attitude to my children has improved, and so yes I think if you get too much engrossed in your professional thing it can leave the emptiness in us ...

There was a personal price to pay for all the effort, which bothered him. He had carried the weekend into the consulting room, which he often did, and he knew it. He was suffering from stress-related illness, and had recently ended up in hospital as a result. But then he was a fortunate man, he said, who never allowed himself to forget whence he came. He was an outsider who had made it on the inside, and this carried its own responsibilities.

6
The Cutting Edge?

Compared with the reality which comes from being seen and heard, even the greatest forms of intimate life – the passions of the heart, the thoughts of the mind, the delights of the senses – lead to an uncertain, shadowy kind of existence unless and until they are transformed, deprivatised and deindivualised, as it were, into a shape to fit them for public appearance. The most current of such transformations occurs in story telling and generally in artistic transposition of individual experiences. But we do not need the artist to witness this transfiguration. Each time we talk about things that can be experienced only in privacy or intimacy, we bring them out into a sphere where they will assume a kind of reality which, their intensity notwithstanding, they could never have had before.

Hannah Arendt, *The Human Condition*

Insiders and Outsiders

Mechthild Hart (1998) works as an academic in a high status, private university in Chicago, and as a volunteer in a public housing literacy scheme in Chicago's inner-city, opposite the university campus. There is a stark contrast between the mostly white middle-class area of the university, with its restaurants, bookshops and diverse facilities, and the poverty, decay and learned powerlessness of the inner-city. In moving between these worlds, Mechthild knows she is, in part, a member of a privileged and dominant social group. She is white, middle class and an academic; she carries within her some of the cultural capital, and power, of the academy. Such signifiers of status make her an insider within the power structure. Yet, she is a foreigner too, with an unusual accent as well as being lesbian. These particular signifiers locate her in a more subordinate position. She is lived diversity and her multiple identities relate, as she terms it, in 'hierarchically organised ways'. As a white, middle-class and university person she can move more or less confidently in a privileged world, sharing and telling its stories. As a lesbian, and foreigner, she is an outsider.

Moreover, her position in the university can alienate her from the world on the wrong side of the street. Her struggle has, in part, been to recover submerged and repressed elements of her story, as a basis for dialogue and shared understanding with some of the peoples of the ghetto; and partly with herself. There are diverse worlds in that self, and she has sought to exploit her 'otherness' as a basis for working with, and learning from, the peoples of the margins. Hart uses standpoint theory to explain her situation and the conflicts engendered in her sense of self. Standpoint theorists argue that we need to see the world from diverse perspectives, across groups and within individual selves. This is not simply a matter of accumulating different knowledge, from different standpoints, and composing a more diverse mosaic. The process is more painful because of a complex power relationship between different identities and knowledge. Hart insists hers is a situation, in these terms, shared by many in the struggle for a better world in which hierarchical relationships – between what is culturally 'inside' and what is 'other', what is acceptable and what is hard to say – can and have to be transcended. And this is to create, in psychological terms, a more integrated and strengthened self with which to engage, more openly, with experience.

Inside Out

GPs in the inner-city, like their patients, have multiple identities. All of us do, in fact. They may, in certain regards, be 'fortunate' men and women, but also aspects of their identity may fit uneasily within the medical lifeworld. Aidene Croft is a foreigner and a lesbian, like Mechthild Hart, and works in a difficult, demanding and impoverished part of London's East End. She is white but talks with a 'different' accent. She mentioned her sexual identity and that this fitted uneasily into the 'male' and predominantly heterosexual culture of medics and training. She was glad to be a representative, in the study, of women and men like her, against the presumption of many doctors, that they are all, or should be, straight, have a heterosexual partner and '2.4 children' at private school. Aidene's experience of being an outsider, as well as emotionally vulnerable, was pivotal to her story.

She was working as a single-hander when we first met, having left a group practice and suffered an emotional breakdown. There were difficulties in her previous practice surrounding money, power and the distribution of work, including who was responsible for the emotional labour of the practice. As she now saw it, difficulties were evident from her initial appointment, alongside, as she freely admitted, her own tetchiness with certain colleagues. The question was raised, from the outset, as to whether the practice staff could cope with her explicit lesbianism, and Aidene thought this a smokescreen behind which some of the partners hid their confused feelings. Yet she also knew the practice needed consensus and partners to work together.

Alternatives

Aidene was taking a course in alternative therapies, when we met for the second time. She had been studying prescriptions:

> ... and out of about fifteen consultations I'd left aside eight sets of notes where I'd used herbs for a consultation. So I'm finding it very useful. I think for a couple of people I'd avoided using drugs that I wouldn't particularly want to start people on – I would have concerns, things like tranquillisers, or starting antidepressants earlier than I otherwise would have. For some people it does the job because it is a short-term reactive process. For other people it gives a breathing space and for things like viruses, flu-like illnesses, recurrent painful ear in children where there is no definite infection, where I can avoid using antibiotics and still send the patient away happy.

She constantly asked herself 'what the hell am I doing here?' in dispensing particular drugs. She could give 'fairly healthy people fairly nasty stuff':

> ... I mean if you're up against the wall with somebody and they're seriously ill and they need the medicine and it's the best one for them, it's great, but in general practice you see a lot of people who don't particularly need it, but there is a lot of pressure to do so as part of the therapeutic process, as part of all sorts of things. Whereas if I had an alternative I could avoid using it while still taking care of the patient.

Aidene was sceptical towards aspects of conventional medicine, for example when she worked in a women's hospital:

> ... and all these doctors were sitting around, completely poo-pooing Pre-Menstrual Tension, that it was only – one of the consultants actually said that it was only something that Sunday Supplement readers ever got, and several of the Asian doctors agreed that nobody in India or Pakistan had PMT! And what kind of ... there wasn't an ovary in the room, shit, you know! So I kind of, at the end, said I don't particularly get PMT you know but I get a bit ratty, a bit of breast tenderness and a bit of this, and I can imagine if you simply multiply that by three, that there are a lot of people very uncomfortable. And I don't think it's anything to do with whether I read the *Guardian* or the *Telegraph*, and there was just this kind of dead silence, and I thought, see what I mean going in the opposite direction – been there all the time – so for my audacity I was given hormone replacement, so I clearly had an interest in these things to present at the next clinical meeting, more or less let's see what you make of that. So I thought,

oh well, they've asked for a show so I'll give them one. So I went off and did all the hormone replacement therapy, all that, and then I gave equal weight to herbs, don't take me wrong, but I looked them up in various common herbal books at the time ... I knew nothing about it: royal jelly and taking calcium and exercise and the evidence was coming out about that then and I came back and gave my presentation and sat back and thought 'Oh God. I wasn't really comfortable doing all this' ... until one of the consultants said well I'm terribly interested in all of this. I've got a very good friend who is a business consultant and executive and she's driven crazy with all these hot flushes ... Suddenly the whole thing turned around and everybody was utterly fascinated with the thought of this.

Personal Roots

We touched, early in the research, on the personal and family roots of her 'alternative' narrative. We talked around the distress in the group practice and she tended, for good reasons, to gloss over it, saying she didn't want to talk about it, and there were problems, in any case, of confidentiality. She cared, still, for her former partners.

Aidene had originally wanted to study microbiology and asked, at school, what a microbiologist did and didn't like what she heard. Somebody suggested she try medicine, and she thought 'they were cracked'. She was in boarding school and saw there were three girls planning a medical career, and getting most attention. She started telling the teachers she was going to be a doctor, and they were soon helping her too:

> ... Maybe that's the root of the thing, I had no idea why, which always made me question – I just knew I had a good brain and I didn't know what to do, so I knew that if I went to school for another six years I would have all kinds of things open to me, ranging from administration, research, psychiatry, paediatrics, you know. I knew that there was a whole – no matter what you wanted to do you could find a role, and a lot of kudos and status, and you know, everybody will be very proud of me and wasn't I very clever and all the rest of it. Everybody – where I come from you know, to be a doctor, to be a teacher, a nurse or a doctor, or a priest, it's more, it's kind of, it's wider than parents. Being a doctor is a big thing.

She described her family background as 'complicated', in early interviews. Her father came from impoverished roots. He had a good brain and worked for the government, and then became an entrepreneur. He was obsessive about education, and half the family (there were many children in 'a good Catholic household') rebelled and the other half conformed, she said. Sometimes the bright ones rebelled and the stupid ones conformed; in her case she conformed, but always with a hint of rebellion.

Picking Up the Pauses

We explored the relationship between her identity and patients:

> You know I think because if your sexuality is outside the normal experience of people's expectations of their doctor, it leads to identification with everybody from Greeks to Turks, black people, Irish people, you know what it's like to be an outsider, you know, to fudge around issues, to not quite explain, for people to instantly lose their curiosity or suddenly go quiet or whatever. All my experience is about being out of orb and extremely positive. You just know that there is that hesitation that people then rethink. You know like when the financial adviser comes. The most recent one was sitting in this room with me you know and says 'What does your husband do?' you know, and I say 'I don't have a husband', and you know, you just move to the next step, 'Hm, right', and then you carry on, no problem ... Last week I was with the guy who does the LIZEI programmes and he had a nine-year-old son and he assumed that I was married or divorced or something, and I said 'No, my partner is a woman and I'm a lesbian' and it was like fine, but it's there, you know that people just have to shift their assumptions a bit. But that's quite nice in a way; it is nice not to be ... it's a mixture. And I think it makes me more accepting of people. A lot of doctors find it terribly difficult to just accept people as they are without trying to change them into the wrong perception, so I think it makes that easier.
>
> ... because being a GP is such an individual art and some people choose doctors who don't pick up the pauses deliberately, because the pauses are too painful ...

Aidene had no idealised view of many of her patients, either. She was more able to empathise with some people, and groups, than others. She could be impatient, she said, with Turkish people who came with no dictionary and no English, and yet had expectations that she was there to solve all their problems. 'They want three housing letters and all the rest of it, I get just as impatient!' She got on well with Afro-Caribbeans, and also with Celtic peoples because their expression and humour were similar to her own. She felt closest to immigrants from the Carribean and Ireland. She understood feelings of loss, and the myth that one day all would be well and they would return home. Being here was always temporary, even if it was for ever. She was sensitive to the mental distress of many minority patients, and wanted to research mental health issues among different populations, '... and if some person like me doesn't do it, why the hell should anybody else, do you know what I mean? – it's like putting something back'.

She talked of how black and Irish people were over-represented in mental health services, but with little understanding, among medics, as to why. Such people are twice as likely to be admitted to hospital than the indigenous white population, with almost every classification of mental illness. She had done research indicating that rates of depression were greater among women than men, but the rates for both sexes in the minority communities exceed those of the 'English'. Rates of schizophrenia were high too, as were a range of anxiety states and personality disorders (Tilki, 1996; Cochrane and Singh, 1989). Alcohol-related problems, and suicide, were higher, and there was also evidence that some immigrant groups were reluctant to access care (AGIY/FIS, 1997).

Racism and Medics

Racism was ubiquitous in medical culture, Aidene said:

> ... All the white doctors were known by their first name, and all the Asian doctors were known as Dr Subamannian, or ... I just called them all by their first name, and eventually all the other doctors started calling them by their first name, so it was Geeta and Mibubu ... It is amazing how something can be so obvious and so just accepted. Whether it was that the white English doctors assumed that the Asian doctors wouldn't want to be known ... but the situation just carries on, and one of the jobs that I went to, the secretary who had been there since the year dot, working with this consultant who was close to retirement age ... She said 'Oh it's so lovely not to have an Asian doctor, for a change', ... and of course all the other doctors were Asian, because it was a geriatric post ...

She was an outsider too:

> ... And I feel a strain and a struggle, simply being different, simply telling stories in a different way. And people just simply not knowing how to listen to stories, not having music around, there are things that are to do with just everyday life, they are not special things ... So what has that got to do with disease? I suppose it's all soul music and food for the soul and if you don't have that it is very easy for the body to ... Well I actually did a survey as part of an audit, and I forget the actual findings but it certainly did show – it bore out the statistic of 60 per cent of ... it actually showed a very high percentage of consultations were about mental health.

Being the outsider could be crucial to doctor–patient relationships. People intuitively knew, one way or another, that, in part, she was one of them:

> I don't divide myself into different people and I'm very much like that with patients. Patients talk about difficulties with children. I'll say 'You know that I understand, I've been there'. I take the kids and cuddle them and say 'Very nice, now you can have them back!' ... So when they have a big crisis it's not – I'm not an edifice, so I think that is what works for me ... I think the biggest thing is that you might not be able to solve all the problems, but why would a doctor want to solve all the problems? Maybe that comes from my background of not going to doctors, you know if I see people and they're not ill and I can't help, I don't keep bringing them back, you know I send them to Citizens Advice and tell them quite firmly that is where they should be directing their energy. Maybe some things I don't take on board – I take on board what I think I can be helpful with and feel fairly easy about closing the door as well.
>
> ... Not infrequently I say to people 'Given that I've left my magic wand at home this is what I can do!' That line I use three or four times a week, which means I have every sympathy for your position, but these are the things I can do but I can't do anything more than that. Whilst still holding you in a sympathetic frame of mind.
>
> ... What I feel I'm doing is listening and filtering out what is the doctor's role, which of course is as long as it is wide. I'm filtering out what I can do and telling the patient that I'll deal with those areas and this is the follow-up. And the rest I understand is very difficult and painful to live with, but I can't address it – I can't make it better.

There is only a certain amount a doctor can do: you can write a letter to the housing department of the local council, she said, but you can't provide the house.

A Developing Conversation

Themes were reworked, and in more depth, over the period of the research, while new ones emerged:

> There is a really interesting theme ... When I started off as a doctor, I think I was just petrified and stunned between my living as, I was going to say, a rampant lesbian. No, a very active, social life and political life and campaigning life, lobbying. Very much as a socialist, feminist, a whole umbrella group dealing with employers, employment issues, day care, abortion, all the things that make up, that actually made up the early Seventies. Very

burning issues. And when I was at medical school they were very separate. That was my person and then I would take the head to medical school. The head: in a motor bike, in leathers, in trousers for my exams and breaking all the images, but still just very much my head and they can take or leave the rest of me. But not really, that wasn't real. It was real in so far as I needed to earn a living, find a role in life. It was real, but ... looking back ... they were very, very separate ... I was very much trying to connect the two ... I couldn't actually tolerate that level of incompatibility.

... I can right this minute remember instances where I felt physically sick at what I witnessed and was powerless to do, I felt powerless. There was a woman who had just given birth to her seventh or eighth child and was told that she had cancer in the middle of a ward round, with about seven or eight people, people in beds next door. She was post-partum. I can remember feeling surreal; it was a feeling of 'Am I the only one?' And of course then you think well everybody else is then off to the next patient. And by the time that you have registered that this actually really happened, somebody is asking you who is this patient, when were they admitted, what were the findings. I found it very difficult to remember all of these facts. So I desperately was trying to survive myself in this culture of mechanisation of people. So that was one instance. And times in that gynae department ... One woman came back from America. She has a coil in. She wasn't married and the minute she went out the door the consultant said 'slut'.

... There was another woman who was told her son had cancer... and the minute the ward round was over I just went and found her down in X-ray, surrounded by strangers, while her kid was having an X-ray to see whether or not he had a kidney tumour ... The kid came in with a UTI, the next minute she is in the middle of a ward round with people being told that it was probably a cancer and we will know in an hour. I remember going down and finding her after the ward round, because it wasn't much to do, but at least I could talk to her, but nobody in training had said it is actually important. Nobody gave any value to that.

A male and conformist ethos enveloped hospitals:

... Well most people are heterosexual give or take varying degrees of comfort or discomfort, but if you get people in a group, like a football club, or a rugby club, or a hospital, or a school, everybody wants to be normal. They want to comform ... Yes, with all that you get all the doctors going out with the nurses and the nurses in their sexy uniform, black tights with seams, you know the stereotypes within it. And you know jack-the-lad. They were all driving MG Midgets and they came with the white coat and stethoscope and the extra dick that you get ... and all the student nurses. So where was

I? Hospitals, they are coming down with lesbian nurses, but they sure as hell weren't knocking on my door ... I think that was because I shut down. I just got so that I walked around with my shoulders up around my ears, not being able to wait until the bell went and I could escape to being a person. So I had left all that and thought well that is me, finished, but I can earn a living ...

A Significant Other

She found more humanity among the GPs she met:

... right, well I am not going to give up completely until I have at least given it a go, because it did seem to have some potential for living like a human being. It was this whole us and them. You are in hospital medicine in order to survive. It has got to be us and them. And 'they' are a permanent nuisance, inconvenience, 'they' being the patients. And I just did not fit in with the hospital. You know hospital is an institution. It has got this whole institutional identity, which I think a lot of it is denial of human experience. Whilst there are extraordinary people working and I worked with some really really good people, the whole culture was alien.

And she forged a strong relationship with a GP trainer:

I had a wonderful trainer, very, very astute, insightful, a really very, very nice man. And thought yes this is it. This is where it is at.
  ... I think the main thing was just having a weekly tutorial, which was just smashing, after years of learning a bit here a bit there, gleaning. Feed me, feed me, this is a fascinating subject. And managing to get attached to a good person here and a good person there, but having to put up with all the crap all around it. Here was this three-hour teaching session ... You could be very honest about your deficiencies in learning. I had done paediatrics and gynae and house jobs. I knew sod all about dermatology ... this was a really clever bloke. I mean clever, clever in a very wide sense. Within two or three weeks I was in there saying – Jesus I haven't a clue about dermatology, give me some pictures, skins, I had no experience of this kind of skin ... I think as well, I had left home when I was sixteen or something. I was one of eleven children and suddenly here I was being given this – I had gone to boarding school, it has always been out of my way, I want that bit of whatever is going. That is mine. And suddenly it was all – 'Now what would you like? Where can we go? What can we do?' So from my experience, coming from that restricted background, it just seemed incredibly generous and useful ... he was somebody who respected people. I could learn from

him that much more and he was a well-established family doctor. He had delivered half of his practice.

For the first time, she felt seen, valued and 'fed' in medicine, as she did in her personal life with a new partner. The trainer accepted and respected her as she was, and made her feel that she could be and do more as a doctor, in her own way. Sean Courtney, in reviewing research into adult learning, noted how frequently a significant other was essential to what he termed 'life spacing': taking risks, experimenting, and managing transitions (Courtney, 1992; West, 1996). Learning, in this view, is a profoundly inter-subjective experience, in which disparate parts of a self and identity may be projected, openly, into the transitional space between people, and if valued and understood by them, can be reinternalised in strengthened ways. If there is, within each of us, a hierarchically ordered struggle between different identities, then resolving it is a social process.

A Breakdown

Her first and major breakdown came, however, after the trainee year. She was married and separated from her husband and moved in with a new partner:

> We had just bought a house, the kids were living with us more and more, so there were fewer custody issues. I had spent all my life struggling and keeping my head kind of just above eye level and suddenly it was like these whole horizons opened up and I went doolally, suddenly couldn't handle it. It was like heh, it was all this Catholic stuff as well, it's about guilt. You have to be suffering to be happy. And suddenly I wasn't suffering any more. I was dead. I swear to God that is the truth. I don't know whether, I very rarely heard other people break down because they were threatened ... People find happiness, happiness is the hardest thing to cope with. Because you are always afraid that someone will take it away. And then you are left with a double disappointment, it is even harder to pull yourself up ... After my child was born, I did become euphoric for several months, which is quite common. Everything gets quite a different focus. It is like you can't see the wood for the trees, the trees are nearer than the grass kind of and I can remember thinking God I hope this doesn't crash ... and my trainer was really helpful. He said you will be fine, just don't push yourself. You haven't got the constitution at the moment. He was really encouraging.
>
> ... Look, where I come from it is called a nervous breakdown. And everybody knows what it is called and what it is and it means that you are not quite with it but you are not mad enough to go ... whatever the local equivalent is. Everybody recognises this concept except doctors. But my

stepmother long ago told me that 'they might know very clever things up in them universities, but keep your feet well on the ground girl because they really don't know it all'.

... It was a life crisis where I was reinterpreting ... I really had grown up thinking that you suffered to exist, suffer the little children, and you don't have today because you put aside for tomorrow ... work is a struggle and everything is a bind and suddenly I am living with this woman who is great, she has just got a house, she was raised in a flat in the East End, she has just got this lovely bay-windowed, semi-detached house, she is thrilled. I have got a career, we have got the kids, we are happy, Jesus what is going to happen tomorrow. So it was a life crisis I would say. And I went to a really nice psychiatrist who said don't be silly, you don't need tablets and you won't kill yourself and you will be fine ... My trainer was wonderful ... I suppose I think that many people are a lot less open about having a breakdown than I am. You know I can feel people being shocked in circumstances where I say – when I had a breakdown a few years ago this was a consequence or whatever ... I feel it is part of my story and I am not going to hide it because it is convenient to other people, makes other people uncomfortable. I suppose I feel that what I am now integrates those experiences. I have put a lot of work into integrating them and not warding them off ... And you are going along and working hard and you know putting your best into everything and it suddenly turns upside down. I mean that was a very profound experience in my life. You are putting your best into something. You think you are getting along with people and it all completely overturns itself on its head. Well I have learned a lot from that. Some of the things I wouldn't have wanted to have learned and many of the outcomes have been extremely positive for me. It has really pushed me into a whole dimension that I may not have explored and given me a lot more confidence. And that reflects very much on how I feel as a woman doctor ...

Washing Patients' Socks

She talked some more about her family of origin towards the end of the research:

... My actual mother died when I was two. Just gone two. So life can't crap from really a bigger height can it? Yes sure, people are starving as well you know but, yes it was tough.

Very very difficult ... I was a very bright, but very socially immature child, which makes sense doesn't it? But I always had this driving force which was probably over-developed because of my circumstances. I knew everything that was going on. So, I mean examples are when I was eleven, no thirteen, we moved to a small village. This was one of the serendipitous things that happen. For the first time in my life I thought I had gone to heaven ... I thought I had died and gone to heaven. I walked to school surrounded by mountains and countryside and I was the kind of teenager who loved poetry and walking along country lanes, but so were a lot of my contemporaries. This wasn't so odd, although it sounds odd now, but this was – we would often go off for walks, we used to cycle, we used to climb, do all those kind of, go swimming. This was not so unusual as it might sound now, so this was perfect for me. In this gorgeous house. My father had decided, he made these arbitrary decisions, he just ended up places where nobody knew where they were going ... So life kind of happened with these major accidents. You were suddenly translocated – 'We are moving next week' – you know.

And I couldn't live at home. Things were just really nervous and edgy at home and I couldn't live at home, so I was the only one that lived away from home while they were at university ... From that, when I went to university then, I had a few clues when I was in boarding school – shit no ... I had grown up in the Catholic sense of sin and mortification and you know, God please, why let me off with being a paraplegic, you know I would just love to be a quadriplegic just to prove how much you love me ... Very powerful imagery. And my mother had died, my step-mother wasn't one's greatest substitute. Life didn't get much, I mean I lived it. You know before I was four I was on to my third mother, so I didn't need any introduction to them and when they said all this I said fine I know all this.

... Then I went to New York and shared an apartment with this absolutely gorgeous, voluptuous, totally energised woman and I just thought, oh God please don't do this to me. Go away, I am not interested. Life is tough enough already. And until I just gradually thought heh this could be fun, what the hell. At least she won't expect me to wash her socks.

... Which led me to offering to wash people's socks. You know how it is.

The Good Things

There was a danger, she said, of forgetting the good parts of being a GP:

I am now having an interview with you, and then I have a busy surgery this evening. Now there will be a couple of patients I could shoot in the middle of that surgery. Two of them will be very aggravating, five of them will have very simple acne-type things, two will be useful interventions and one I will go 'phh', nice one.

... I did an eight-month check yesterday, with a baby who is arching and scissoring and has abnormal tone. They have a sibling with severe multiple congenital abnormalities, and I feel terrible about the consultation. I have now got to refer this child ... for further developmental assessments and I am very worried that there is something wrong, but I feel satisfied that I did a good job. I had nothing, the mother was reporting no problems and of course she wouldn't because her older child is severely disabled. She doesn't know what a normal child is, so I feel dreadful about it. I wish it wasn't me. I wish I didn't find that, but I feel like I've done my job well and that early intervention with physio, or with whatever may lead to, you know, positive outcomes or whatever.

... Yes there was one patient, there was a death, suicide of a mother, this was the grandmother and there was this tragedy of this baby. This was what the patient was presenting, that this baby's mother had died and the family were left with this total tragedy ... but there was this real sense of tragedy in the whole room ... There was no redeeming or rescuing factor, and we really got into this tragedy big time and I said well wait a minute – is there nothing about this – and of course there is this baby, very, very live baby. Having a baby ... a tragedy? ... It was an enormous tragedy, but there was a whole sort of future.

... I think this job is very privileged in sharing other people's journeys ... A patient, I can picture a particular patient. She has just come back pregnant with her second one and she says – 'God, can I cope?' 'Can you cope?' 'I think I will be better this time.' 'I am sure you will. It never gets any scarier.' And we laugh ...

The secret was being authentic:

... being myself in my job ... has grown so that when I see people, we are two people, and yes I have enormous power over their lives, 'enormous power', in great big bloody inverted commas. But I have enormous kind of ritualistic power in their lives. They are going to their doctor and I am the doctor in their imagination. That role is what I am inhabiting. But I know I am me ... so when they walk in it's very straightforward, well knowing that I am part of that ritual, am part of that role in society and actually very down to earth. You know the patients who get used to me and like my style we get along very matter of factly. So I don't try and fit into that mythical role and they very quickly learn that they can come and ask me to do something and I will either say yes or no, or that's possible, or let's try this, or whatever.

... A lot of medicine is to listen with the story and to intervene when it is appropriate for medicine to intervene ... I think that there are points that you can intervene. There are some times when you say to people – I think you should give up smoking and you know that they can't ... whereas other times there is a window of opportunity, when you can actually communicate with people. You can actually look them in the eye and say – you must give up smoking. You know. There's times, it is often not what you say, it is the point of communication that is important ... you don't need evidence to help people get themselves better, unless what you are using is toxic and harmful. It changes the whole balance and the vast majority of things that people get sick with, that go to the GP, are things that make them feel them unwell, many of which are the result of the lifestyle and lack of understanding and the crap food and the cigarettes ... People feel uncomfortable enough and often they want some guidance and I can probably make them a lot more comfortable ... So this is a gender issue. This is, women and mothers all over the world saying, you know, my son is not well enough to go to work and he is only twenty-three. What is the matter with him? This is 'women speak' and I have got a nephew who is completely bolloxed, you know what I mean. And there isn't anybody who would actually sit down and speak to him. Even though he goes to psychologists, there is nothing integrated. You are either physically sick, in which case you have everything examined from head to foot, or you are psychologically sick, in which case you are a dustbin case ... What I got fed up with was being there to dole out quite toxic prescription drugs, without any patient understanding.

... Being myself has relieved me of the burden of the whole hierarchy of medicine. That I could just be the particular doctor that I am, with that particular patient. The rest of it was completely immaterial.

Diversity in Practice

Aidene had learned to work eclectically:

My first paradigm of using complementary medicine is to limit damage. I think a lot of the things that we use are actually damaging to the human system ... like the use of steroids or the use of antibiotics, this has all hit the media, which is very nice for me because I have been doing this for years, even before I got involved in complementary medicine I was very wary of valium. I always hated valium even in the Seventies and stood up in lectures or whatever and said that I have my doubts about them. Because they are just so potent. It is like using a sledgehammer to dampen down everything in the human system. So using complementary medicine I manage to avoid using them as nuts to crack, as a sledgehammer to crack a nut. I do use them as a sledgehammer to crack something worthy of a sledgehammer. I mean if somebody has cellulitis, ascending cellulitis, from a severe infection, I am the first person to put somebody on antibiotics, bloody large doses for as long as it takes.

... I wouldn't claim that complementary medicine has all the answers for all people, under all circumstances, at all times. But it has many answers for most people in a gentler way for much of the time, which I think is very relevant to general practice. In fact I think it would also be very relevant if wider facilities were made available. It goes back to doctors divorcing themselves from nursing. How can we expect people to get better without adequate nursing? But the whole of medical services, it seems to me now, is about managing machines to manage health and ignoring the role that food and housing and wider welfare has on people's lives ... I think the population has realised that and is turning to complementary practitioners in their millions.

There were two final threads in her story: on gender and the personal roots of professional beliefs:

I was aware when I was in the group practice that there were gender issues but I can remember being shouted down for even suggesting it and going home and thinking – whoops, well they were not very comfortable with that. I could work with the things that I was aware of without vocalising them. So I just knew not to vocalise them. I just worked my way around them. But they were very upset that I would suggest that there were gender issues at play. 'How can you say that?' 'Well I am just saying it.' 'Well prove it.' 'How can you prove it?' And yet I feel the turning point within the practice, looking back with years of hindsight now, the turning point was not accepting the established hierarchy within the practice ... Refusing to accept the dominant ideology in its entirety ... I mean one of the staff was unhappy with the situation involving one of the partners and the initial analysis was that she was unhappy with her job and wanted, what is the word, constructive dismissal. I didn't accept this analysis of the circumstances and sorted it out and the partner ended up apologising, but I think by being challenging, and not accepting the status quo it set me up when I was ill for then being dispensable, but because I am a bit uncomfortable to be around anyway.

... It is very difficult ... It is not easy to analyse and I think when we are now working at this level of professional involvement with men it is not that people are being crass, it is not that people are doing the obvious things that you would find on a factory floor ... a lot of it has to do with being nice. Being a nice lady doctor, who is nice to the patients and who everybody goes to for their emotional fix. That is part of it. Watching out for the staff, knowing what is going on in the office dynamics. The thing with the member of staff was a good example. You know one partner ... knew 'management speak' and it is a very male organisational hierarchical structure ... and there was a direct clash because he was there saying 'Well

I think this is constructive dismissal, as an employee.' ... Is this June we are talking about? June has worked here for God knows how many years ...

No doubt other partners could tell other stories about the group practice. But the gendered assumptions structured into the everyday world of medicine were a recurring theme across many of the narratives. Aidene finished her story by revisiting part of her childhood:

> ... As a child I just always loved plants and gardening ... We had gardens, but you know they were not terribly well kept. But from the time that I first had access I was trying. I loved biology, I loved botany. I was given a lot of praise for being very good at it. We moved to the country when I was thirteen and I thought, this is it, I have moved to paradise. I thought this was a great step forward compared to city living. All of it was kind of like completing a circle. Going back to why I actually started medicine, which was because I thought there can't be anything more fascinating in the whole world. And various threads to do with looking for yourself if you have big problems of neediness. I think people find medicine because it covers their own neediness. And there is one place that you are going to be vulnerable, that you are terrified of being vulnerable, it is being sick. So you protect yourself by looking after sick people. Totally neurotic. Not a total bunch of neurotics, but I think probably higher than average.

One physician healing herself; past and present became merged. Many people, she insisted, had lost faith in the conventional orthodoxies. For patients with chronic diseases, like migraine and irritable bowel or asthma, they may take the medication but it doesn't work, and they continue to live with the symptoms. There are alternatives but people are not informed. Aidene took me to the gendered as well as the intimate heart of medicine, and into the struggle to be a more authentic doctor and person.

Starting Points

Dr Daniel Cohen, like Aidene, feels an outsider in medicine. His big crisis came eight years ago:

> ... I think I expressed a great deal of distress at that time of what do you do if you're working nine sessions a week as a GP, plus lots of on-call, very, very hard, and you're having no time for extra training, no time for reflection.
> ... The scale of the work and the endlessness of it. The scale being that you can go in at eight in the morning and be dealing with people's pain continually without a break and go on till seven or eight in the evening: to

a degree and with a volume that I think is almost inconceivable for most other outsiders. There are very few professions which have got any sort of an analogous workload in terms of its volume or its intensity. But also the endlessness in that there isn't any clear career development – let's say for somebody in their late thirties who finds themselves in that position: you know a hospital consultant can possibly look forward to increasing managerial power and less clinical involvement as they get older. Other professions have got their hierarchical structures. For a GP there is no obvious evolution from that point, which you may reach at age thirty-seven to thirty-eight. So the point at which you're expecting to retire is in another thirty-plus years, twenty-plus years' time.

Daniel went into psychotherapy for a time and trained as a therapist too:

I think I feel less stressed by the clinical work, although it's hard to tell how much of that just results from doing less of it and how much results from having a more therapeutic stance.

... I mean I am less likely to get overwhelmed by the stuff that comes through the door, I think I am able to sit back and leave responsibility in the hands of the patients I'm dealing with ... It was something that had been around for years and years ... So when I decided to take a sabbatical, one obvious option was to complete my training ... That was why I chose it, but in a way it could have been another kind of therapy. I think it might have had exactly the same consequence. I think the essence of it is that it gave me time for personal development and for reflection.

Questions of self, families, and the cultural roots of many anxieties, were inseparable from his work as a GP. There was no neat distinction between questions of 'Who am I?' or 'Where do I come from?' or 'Why do I have the kind of problems that I think I have?' and those such as 'Why am I doing my work – what is the nature of my work?' 'How can I best help the people I'm working with – what is the nature of their problems?' There was a seamless web connecting the doctor to patients, their story to his. Daniel's inner world consisted of a series of conversations involving many characters. There was the heroic GP who could solve everything. There was the consumerist patient, who might also be part of the doctor, who said 'I've read about this thing and I'm as informed as you are and I want it.' There was the sceptic who insisted that GPs had little time. Sometimes one character might predominate, at other times, another. The characters shifted in significance, and each might need to enter the dialogue, at a particular moment. Two patients might say of the same drug 'I demand it because I've heard it's a miracle drug' and 'How dare you give this to me? I've read that it causes cancer in rats.' They might have been talking about the same drug, but have read different newspapers that morning or heard different accounts on the radio. Every consultation had its cast of characters and conflicting stories, within the doctor as well as the patient. It was a question of living with the diversity, and learning, empathically, how to respond in the moment.

Wanting to Be a Psychiatrist

Daniel never intended to be a GP and imagined himself as a psychiatrist or a psychoanalyst. But during medical training he felt alienated, even repulsed by institutional psychiatry and simply could not see himself working within 'NHS mental health culture'. He was drawn towards paediatrics, which he thought a discipline combining feelings, including gentleness, with technical and medical expertise. But he kept failing exams. He had a poor grasp of the technical detail needed, for instance, to be a neonatal paediatrician. You had to be a very good thinking scientist, he said, which he definitely was not. He loathed the way psychiatry was practised:

> It's just a ghastly environment. I didn't like the sort of detached way in which psychiatrists dealt with their patients, I didn't like the sort of pseudo-medical stance that they took. It sort of screams at you out of the pages of Ronnie Laing, and it hasn't changed. I think that psychiatrists and psychiatric nurses within institutions largely treat patients in the sort of objectifying manner that Charcot sort of demonstrated with his hysterics. And I think it's sort of obscene really. And it's extraordinary how little that's changed. And essentially I think the main purpose of institutions ought to be as asylums literally – of just places that give people bed and breakfast while they recover. And yet there is this sort of illusion of making interventions, which are often, I think quite dehumanising.

General practice offered, in comparison, more humanity:

> ... I think that general practice is at the feminine end of a masculinised culture. I think general practice has always been more touchy/feely, although it is looking over its shoulder the whole time to keep up its street cred with the real blokes in the hospitals.

But there was a paradox:

> ... I am aware of two simultaneous processes going on at the moment in a kind of dialectic. One is a hyper-masculinisation of the profession in terms of, let's say, the formation of primary care groups and the grasping of power by GPs as a profession and the idea that GPs will actually run the health service on the one hand, and on the other hand a development of a much

more reflective stance among a minority of GPs, but I still think it is the minority actually. I am in touch with a network of various people around the country involved in different projects or organisations or interest groups who are almost pulling in an opposite direction from the political trend towards masculinisation, and I have a feeling that that's a dialectic which has always existed and will always exist and that the battle isn't, as it were, lost or won, or can it be or should it be, but it just continues. And certain people like myself will identify themselves with the 'feminine' position and certain people won't.

... I suppose a great deal of my job is masculine, perforce. I mean as we were trying to start this interview it was interrupted by a phone call from hospital with information as to whether a patient did or did not carry a particular germ. I suppose that intrusion irritated me like all intrusions irritate me into a process that I would much rather was more reflective, but I have to deal with it and it is my job to deal with it whatever else is going on. And a lot of the job, all day every day, has to accept that those are the conditions in which one works to be a modern doctor. The feminine side is that I am constantly striving to contain and manage those sorts of moments in order to create space for feminine types of experience to be possible. So that I would, largely speaking, manage to work in an environment where I am not likely to get many phone calls of that sort and not to get drawn into the kind of omnipotent theatre that a lot of doctors get drawn into where the phone is ringing every ten seconds to impress everybody else and let them know how important they are.

The feminine? Yes. Acceptance, tolerance, understanding of process rather than events and outcomes, sorts of things that are fluid rather than things that are chopped up and categorised. A sense of connection and of connection being more important than anything and of values being more important. I am trying to remember an aphorism to do with being in the moment rather than looking for some kind of triumphalist crock of gold at the end of the rainbow really.

A patient came to mind:

... she had an illness of rather mysterious cause and she needed medication for it and a referral to a psychiatric nurse, all of which I facilitated in quite a sort of agency-type way, in the hope and the expectation that if I stuck with her through this and continued to see her once a month, ostensibly for a review of her medication, that things would emerge and inevitably after many months have passed she is able to actually reframe what she has gone through in terms of a highly unsatisfactory marriage which she wasn't really able to face up to before. She is able to see in a way that she in some way needed the illness to give her time out and to give her time to reflect on this. And she is gradually sort of reconceptualising what has happened in terms of a need to challenge her husband to do some work at their relationship or to get out … has now on her own initiative come off the anti-depressants, is looking at the possibilities of counselling and therapy – so that I suppose I have accepted the constraints of a world in which people expect and demand to be diagnosed and medicated in the interests of what I see as a more important long-term project which is actually to explore new meaning in their lives.

'Patient-centred medicine', Daniel said.

Recovering Roots

Daniel had been involved in recovering different parts of his identity, over a long period, and this was an aspect of wider cultural change:

… and finding to my astonishment really that being Jewish and the child of refugees who had fled from Nazism was actually a hugely important part of my identity. Something which sounds absurd now, it was something that had never even crossed my mind, that it might be an important part of who Daniel Cohen was. I had been brought up with a lot of ideas about assimilation and that ethnicity and culture was something you chose rather than something that you arrived with and had to manage and it was sort of therapy that led me to a review of all of that really and to an understanding that I couldn't, I couldn't shrug it off. I had to kind of go into it rather than leave it.

… there is something that is going on in the much wider community … I think that for ten, twenty, thirty years after the war the community of refugees was utterly traumatised by what they had experienced, and also out of necessity completely focused on material survival, on doing well, rebuilding their businesses, on their children being properly educated etc. and there was suddenly a burgeoning among people of my generation in the late Seventies, early Eighties, of a curiosity about where we had come from and challenging our parents, or the parental generation about the way they had dealt with their experiences and so there has been a massive kind of 'outing' if you like, of the second generation of refugee children and a massive return to the community and to religion. But I also think there has been a focus on ethnicity and a pride in ethnicity that has also surfaced in the wider community around the same time. And it has obviously been happening with Afro-Caribbean people. It has obviously been happening with Muslims. There are a lot of communities where people, who were actually quite ashamed about their origins in the Sixties and Seventies, are actually now fiercely proud of it and finding some way to express it. And I think what happened to the Jewish community was part of the wider collective reowning of ethnicity.

His growing spiritual beliefs were part of the same process. Towards the end of an interview Daniel said:

> ... I was having a conversation with myself at one point about why am I not bringing in more of – one particular dimension of my life which is very much connected with my wife, who is a minister of religion, I don't know if you're aware my wife is doing this, and so I have a third job as a minister's spouse, and it is actually enormously important to me and it affects my work in all sorts of ways. And I was actually asking myself at one point why I wasn't bringing that into play, so it was interesting I, by Freudian slip, I phoned her at the beginning of this interview! Clearly wanting to bring her in some way, and I suppose that is the most feminine and feminised of all the different kinds of aspects of my work. And it is work, I mean I go as a spouse to her congregational events and so on. So there is all of that, that I was sort of hovering on the edge of what I was saying and didn't quite come in.

We shared thoughts about spirituality and 'God' in the consultation:

> If I can use the theological language it was actually about creating God, it was not there to describe God or try and convince oneself of God as an external objective, and rather punitive power, but that actually this was about reviving, sustaining and the constant continuous creation of God. I suppose it is about sort of perceiving oneself as a participant in continuous creation, which cannot be about reason. It can only be about values and meaning and conviction and an act of faith, of actually saying this will only happen if I will it to happen. That it is a matter of making it for oneself, making God for oneself.
>
> ... I think it sustains me here because I think to try and do a job like this, especially the clinical side of the work, in the absence of a value framework, I think would be suicidal. And I don't think it terribly matters how one labels that value framework and I know people, and work with people, who I think have a deeply religious stance, but might call it socialism, or humanism, or whatever. I don't think that matters. But I think the other way I would say it affects me is that I think at the most difficult, and also the best moments of general practice, I think one is operating, I am

operating from what I would call a spiritual base rather than a purely technical base, and there are moments when you actually know that what is really at stake is moral rather than medical and the engagement with people has to be moral rather than medical.

... I am referring to those moments in general practice where in a consultation you start off by thinking what you are doing here is facilitating, almost technical, rational decisions about what you should recommend or what the patient should choose. And suddenly you realise that you are engaged with somebody jointly in a sort of desperately important struggle about how to be good, how to be real, how to make a choice which is right and it's often to do with life and death. It is often to do with sort of birth, marriage and dying. I become aware that the sort of paraphernalia of medicine and prescriptions and operations and referrals and all of that is really a kind of lower order manifestation really of something which is spiritual.

... I love the idea that here is a community, a collection of people, that is simply about values. It has no other purpose except to further a set of moral and religious values. It is not there to produce anything. There is no outcome. There's nothing to market, there's nothing to be audited. It is simply about pure value and pure meaning and I find that very anchoring. And it is a great relief. Maybe that is something else about being there as a spouse, also it's not my responsibility to give, that I can receive in that context as well ... It was something that was totally absent until I was in my mid-thirties – completely. I think the great shock for a lot of people of our generation, was, I was certainly brought up with the assumption, that religion would be dead and gone by the time I reached middle age and that no self-respecting, intelligent person would have any involvement with it, whatsoever. And I treated it more or less with contempt. I was brought up to treat it with contempt and it was sort of one of the bigger shocks of my life, maybe the biggest shock, to find myself kind of almost embarrassingly flirting with it in my early thirties and completely won over by it by my mid-thirties. Both in terms of a need for a community of people sharing my origins and traditions, identifying myself with, which I suppose is a kind of ethnic or cultural need, but also the search for some meaning and values that were sort of wider than material ones ... it has happened since I have been in this practice ... and it was a big shock to my partners who have largely remained agnostic or militantly atheist ... that is something that I have had to negotiate. They see me going from a fairly sort of bog standard, liberal, semi-Marxist atheist, to the husband of a minister in the course of ten to fifteen years and have had to understand that that didn't change me in its essence and that they could live with me with my new identity.

The Personal and the Professional

Daniel also rooted his work and beliefs in family history:

> ... I guess this was terribly important ... I think the children of refugees from Nazism were left with existential puzzlement, which is I suppose to do with the meaning of evil and healing and I think it has led enormous numbers of us into caring professions, I mean not necessarily medicine but also social work, therapy, counselling etc. etc. It is an industry that's sort of largely populated by Jewish people, often from refugee backgrounds. So I think it was a very powerful influence although I don't think I realised that at the time. I think it expressed itself as I wanted to sort myself out and understand more about myself and therefore getting, well, my original aim which was actually to become a psychiatrist, would be a way of doing that and then through a process I didn't end up in that discipline, but I think that the sort of wish to heal is always directed at oneself primarily.
>
> ... There are all kinds of different experiences. Firstly my parents were refugees rather than survivors, which makes a considerable difference. A lot of members of their families remained behind and were murdered. But they themselves, their experience was very positive because they got out and for that reason, for example, they were tremendously patriotic about Britain which they perceived as sort of having rescued them. And also they belonged to a group; they had a style of managing it which was simply not to talk about it, and again there are varieties of response. Some people in my position were brought up with their parents talking about absolutely nothing else. I was brought up with it not being talked about at all and then there is the question of whether it was dealt with by religion or by rejecting religion, so there is a lot of pluralism within the way families dealt with it. But I think the unspoken imperative to succeed and not to rebel was very powerful. I don't think I had anything that could remotely be described as an adolescence. I think I was just sort of completely studious and privately very distressed and outwardly tremendously successful, like hundreds of Jewish teenagers I knew.

The 'personal' entered the professional, sometimes in surprising ways. A Somali woman refugee came to the surgery one day:

> ... A Somali family, a mother and five children, father not in this country, possibly alive, possibly not, I don't know. They don't know. May still be alive in Somalia or may have been killed in the war there. May have succeeded in emigrating somewhere else, but hasn't been able to contact the family. Children with a huge range of problems from asthma to epilepsy,

mother speaking very, very little English so that either one of the children translates inadequately, but it is inadequate having a child translate for their mother in the best circumstances. Often just turning up out of the blue without an appointment, needing three or four people to be seen. And the anxiety and the sort of tension that arrives with that sort of situation is absolutely massive for a GP. And yet, at the same time, I am reproaching myself and thinking my God if it is massive for me what is it like for them? And I have a sort of political and a religious and a personal imperative to provide an exceptional service for people like that, but with the fear of what is it doing to me. And I struggle to create situations where I can meet more of their needs really by putting an hour aside for them at a special time with an interpreter. Then they might not turn up and I will be sitting there with the interpreter and the patients haven't come. I have sort of erected this thing which means a lot to me, and actually it doesn't fit with their needs which are immediate and urgent and they can't, how can they, have the least inkling about what the pressures are on me given the urgency of their needs ... The mother of that family brought me a goat's skin rug for Christmas. Somebody had come over from Somalia with this rug and she brought it to me as a gift and I was immensely moved because firstly they are not wealthy at all and secondly it was a really strong symbol that we were providing something, that actually we are a secure base basically and that she identified me as one white British person in authority who she can trust, I hope, and that relates to my own experience as a child of refugees, because my own parents were refugees and I can remember how incredibly important the GP was to us as a secure base. And the other moving thing was that I did succeed recently in getting a long consultation with the whole family with a link worker present. A very, very intelligent link worker who is a Somali doctor herself, but can't practise here so she works as a link worker. And we ended up having the most extraordinary conversation with the mother about Darwinian evolution in relation to why were her children getting asthma and eczema here when children didn't get it in Somalia, and we talked about the way the immune system might be adapted for one environment but actually then is mal-adapted to another environment because the sort of ancestral immune system as it evolved is not to meet what it meets here. And I found myself having a grown-up conversation with this mother of the sort I might have with you and she was transformed from being a sort of exotic stereotype into actually being a sort of intelligent equal. And again that was terribly moving because I felt it was part of, part of a process of becoming a person again, for her. That she could actually have what I would guess is her first conversation with somebody British which wasn't just about immediate needs, about housing or benefits, or prescriptions and that sort of stuff but actually recreate her as an equal adult.

He had never made the connection before, he said. There were differences, for sure, in that his parents were central European Jews who actually chose to have a central European Jewish refugee for their GP. And yet:

> ... I guess he represented to them a kind of bridge and also an aspiration of what they might become and of actually developing lives and careers here. And there was a sort of emotional texture of visits to the doctor which I now very much identify as being about safety and about containment. I use the word secure base in a sort of technical as well as its common-sense meaning of actually being a place to get looked after and a dependable place.
>
> I remember a therapist saying he would be deeply suspicious of any doctor or psychiatrist who wasn't in the job principally to make themselves better. That if you are not on a kind of journey, trying to understand yourself and make yourself whole then you are probably a bit messianic and so I think that is at the heart. And I hope that as a sort of spin-off of that other people get helped as well. I think the best moments are when you get distracted from your preoccupation with making yourself better and can actually can lose yourself in the whole business of empathy with other people, but I think it is in a way always coming back to the business of a personal search, actually trying to find out what life is about and what you should be making of it.

Initial Training, Lifelong Learning

We finished by reconsidering medical training, and the position of the outsider:

> ... remedial therapy for the selective brain damage of doctors ... which is doing the work years afterwards when people are sort of you know, recovering doctors. So I have absolutely nothing to say whatever about undergraduate medical education. I admire the people who dare to get involved, but I feel I would be corrupted by it. I can remember people at my medical school who were psychoanalysts or sociologists who were subversive voices and they were mocked, treated with contempt, given lousy places in every sense in the building, in the curriculum, in people's esteem and I don't perceive that that has changed very much and I don't want to be harmed by it. I don't sort of feel strong enough to go and tackle the establishment in that way. I think it requires very special people to go in with the 'subversive you' and hold on to it in that context ...
>
> ... I don't know how you go into a system where you know kids, and they are kids who have basically come out of a lecture on the dephosphorilation of ATP which they have to know about and then somebody like me comes

in and talks about Foucault and knowledge as power and postmodern deconstructions of knowledge and relativism and the structure of scientific revolutions. I mean I don't know if that is possible or to be honest I don't even know if it is desirable, because there is an argument that says – let them learn this stuff, they need it, you know. You and I need to see doctors who know how many valves there are in a heart and how they all work, what they all do, and what happens when they go wrong and how they go wrong and how they can be corrected. Actually people need to learn that in an environment where they are allowed ... and it can be available years down the line if they want to actually say well you know had you thought of taking on board that people did not always believe it was like this and that extrapolated from history it is perfectly possible that people will see things very, very differently in fifty or a hundred years time in ways that we are not even capable of imagining because we are culture-bound and what difference does that make to your practice and what difference should it make to your practice? But I think to try and combine that kind of message with a truth discourse is highly problematical.

Daniel thought general practice represented the cutting edge of medicine:

... Well, I think in the last five to ten years the medical discourse in the journals and education and so on has been utterly, utterly dominated by the idea of evidence-based medicine to the point, I think, of absolute oppression as if there was nothing except evidence. And to some extent it had to be like that because there was so much sort of sloppy and impressionistic practice going on and somebody had to say, 'Hang on, we have to look at what works', and counting it and seeing that people are actually behaving in a vaguely rational fashion. However, that whole kind of evidence-based culture has existed in a sort of vacuum that ignored the very, very exciting things that were going on in the humanities, in the therapies, in anthropology and sociology and so on where people were beginning to think in new ways about people's lives, and about narrative. I mean the post-postmodernism if you like. We are moving on from postmodernism to something that was about constructing stories. And I think that what has happened in the last couple of years is that there have been enough people around who knew something about both cultures to draw them together. And I think people are now beginning to see that it is not such a polarisation as it appeared to be. That actually evidence may make sense as part of a narrative and the challenging question becomes how do you incorporate evidence into a narrative, rather than, there is no such thing as evidence without a context. So how do you bring evidence to bear in what is essentially an overarching narrative context? Now I have an imaginary real doctor in my head, who is not me, who is saying well narrative is the sloppy end of the market. I mean the kind of doctors who will be interested in narrative are those who can't really understand evidence. But I think there is going to be some kind of synthesis whereby each of us will have to learn to speak the other's language.

... The medical model will continue to be immensely powerful. It will continue to be the dominant paradigm. I mean we are not going to shift, just too much invested in it. It will probably increase its dominance particularly with sort of molecular genetics on the horizon. But I think that it will never be able to overthrow its critique, because it comes from such a narrow epistemology that however powerful it is in practical terms it can't sort of get outside itself in the way that the social sciences can and therapy can. So there will always be a place for very, very powerful critiques.

... Medicine is sort of incapable of reflecting on its own nature. You need something else outside medicine to do that. Molecular genetics can produce incredible outcomes, but it can't think about itself. You actually need outsider/insiders to be able to do that.

... Well I think general practice is the cutting edge. I mean for me the cutting edge isn't more and more of the latest evidence. For me the cutting edge is how to, how to tame that evidence, which isn't to sort of neutralise it, but actually to make it fit with people's lives rather than getting so upset by it that you don't hear people's stories when they come through the door ... It is to be able to use, to offer the evidence to give people intelligent options to incorporate in their own narratives really rather than saying you know you have got to come off your Ventolin inhaler and use Becotide because that is what all the research is showing. It is how to develop those kinds of conversations. It also depends on the patients wanting those kinds of conversations because of course you get patients coming in through the door and saying 'For goodness sake be a doctor and give me something.'

If this represented a compromise with truth, it was nonetheless positive:

I mean if you only see it as an intellectual compromise in the negative sense then you couldn't do the job. I think it is really very similar to diplomacy, diplomats couldn't do their job if they saw compromise as something tawdry. Peace treaties come unstuck, consultations can come unstuck, and diagnosis can come unstuck. I mean I have got some lovely anecdotes now. You know a patient came to me with a problem and the first question I asked was – what do you think it is yourself? And she said – 'Yes my friend said you always say that.' You know in a very kind of bored, resigned voice as if – 'I don't know if I am ever going to get a diagnosis out of you doc.'

Yet he also despised aspects of the mainstream:

> ... I don't believe in what I think the mainstream believes in. If I go to a lecture at a postgraduate medical centre by a local consultant on a main-line subject, something I almost never do these days, I am actually appalled by the discourse, just appalled by it. I mean I am appalled by the whole set of assumptions about the nature of reality, about the assumption of the doctor's power and the assumption of sexist and racist and God knows what else ideas and the assumption, the collusion around that and the idea that that is sort of shared and the lack of reflection on it. I feel profoundly alienated by it, which is why I have so little to do with it.
>
> ... Like mining a seam of gold called the medical fact ... from a sort of pile of shit, which is the patient's sort of life. That is putting it very bluntly and very brutally but I am sure you know what I mean. It is a way of talking about, describing patients, describing patients as if the patient isn't there, and it can operate at any level. I mean at its crassest it is actually saying you know this woman, and it usually is a woman, walked into my consulting room and with enormous effort I discovered what the problem really was, but at the more subtle level it can be just sort of talking about knees as if they weren't attached to anybody. Just talking about symptoms and signs as if they were disembodied, or just objects and the whole of the discourse that goes on around that. Talking about a patient with acute renal failure as if there is not a family around that person who are terrified that the patient is going to die and that they are going to be lost and that that person is a friend, a parent, a child, a lover, workmate, the whole way that that is spoken without adequate respect really to the context.
>
> ... And yet I practise within a very, very orthodox profession. I mean I haven't gone off and become a psychotherapist, let alone an acupuncturist or homeopath or fringe practitioner. So I am an insider in the social sense. Who could be more of an insider than the local GP, but I am very much an outsider in my stance towards it.

GPs were situated between the truth discourse of the mainstream and the uncertainties and messiness of whole people, living in a harsh environment. A subversive synthesis was required, taking what was essential from the medical model but locating this within a person and narrative-focused practice. GPs had to learn how to live on such an edge, on their own terms; the personal and professional were all of a piece.

7

Gendered Practice

... there is a deeper and more significant struggle taking place ... [which is] experienced daily many, many times at all stages of both her professional and wifely concerns. Not only is she impelled to divide her time and energy to cover both home and work, but unlike the male professional, she is constantly beset with divided loyalties, a sense of guilt and often a shaky sense of identity.

Alexandra Symonds, 'The Wife as the Professional'

A Gendered Edge: 'How Things Are Done Round Here'

If feminism and the new politics of identity have challenged traditional, rigid and biologically determinist stories of gender, and have created space within the culture for women and men to experiment with their identities, this is not without uncertainty and continuing inequalities. Caring, of whatever kind, remains undervalued and, in many contexts, continues to be 'women's work'. This chapter focuses on the stories of three women GPs with family responsibilities, including taking care of children at times of difficulty in their careers. The stories illuminate mixed and painful feelings over priorities as between jobs and family and the divided loyalties evoked. The chapter raises fundamental questions about the status and distribution of emotional labour within medicine (and more widely), as well as in the private sphere of the family.

Aidene Croft described how the woman doctors often performed the 'motherly' duties, and yet were castigated if this was challenged. Women were 'mothers' at work as well as at home while the 'father' was more often than not emotionally absent. Workplace culture, as Janet Newman (1999) has described, is often deeply gendered in its everyday practices and in the stories people tell to each other about 'how things are done round here'. Aminatta Forna (1999) observes that it is fashionable to subscribe to the view that men and women have achieved much greater equality at work and in other public spheres, including the significant advances of many women in the labour market, over the last twenty years. However Forna insists this is 'a veneer of equality' which disguises continuing and significant fault lines.

Forna argues that precious little has changed in the division of some domestic responsibilities, in particular child rearing. She quotes a survey by the Family Policy Studies Centre in 1996, which indicated that childcare remained overwhelmingly a maternal affair. Men and women, alike, continue to regard 'mother' as the central player in children's lives. It is she who continues to make the major sacrifices in career terms, regardless of professional responsibilities. The mystique of motherhood – that in some sense she is unique, biologically determined and irreplaceable – retains a powerful discursive grip. If the 'wife' role has loosened somewhat, over three decades, and 'she' is not supposed to be there – greeting her husband with tea or whisky and soda – childcare responsibilities still remain predominantly hers. This can apply equally to professional women with pressures worsening in the greedy, needy environment of contemporary work.

There is, almost certainly, a psychological price to pay for many women. Llewelyn and Osborne (1990) argue that if a woman chooses a particular career and makes every effort to pursue it, it is the rare woman who does not have to modify or alter her plans in response to overt or covert pressure from family, employers and colleagues. Even when women are not planning to have children, they can be seen as potentially more unreliable, treated as future mothers and, in effect, therefore, temporary or part-time workers. Llewelyn and Osborne note that even highly motivated and well-paid professional women (like doctors) are likely to take prime responsibility for domestic and family chores. Some will try, as a consequence, to don the mantle of superwoman, performing a double shift without apparent effort. But the price can be guilt, exhaustion and rage, however repressed; and sometimes a divided, fragile identity. Doctors Sarah Cotton and Claire Barker know the price.

There are, however, other stories to tell as gendered assumptions are being challenged in particular relationships, and in the wider politics of gender. Dr Jane Kelly is pursuing a diverse medical career while her male partner is training to be a counsellor and takes prime responsibility for their two young children. He suffered redundancy and the loss of a traditional public role but survived to rebuild his life in a different way, with more emphasis on relationships, children and the quality of emotional life. Jane considers herself to be more 'masculine' than he, as she progresses in her career, including being a key player in a new Primary Care Group, as well as working for a hospice. Hers is a story of our time too.

Guilt in the Middle

Sarah Cotton has two young children, for whom she is the prime care-giver. She sometimes felt stretched to the limit by the practice, and the area in which she worked, made worse, in the course of the research, by the illness of her young son. She described, early on, doctoring in the inner-city. More patients were struggling with financial, social and psychological problems that tended, as she saw it, to get 'dumped on general practice'. Care had left the community and individuals often had nowhere else to go but to their GP. Yet she was aware too of the limitations of what could be done when problems were more a product of social than individual pathology.

Her practice 'had more patients than ever' who were taking anti-depressants and a growing number of schizophrenics. The practice was responsible for two hostels in the local community catering for mentally ill patients, and a hostel for disturbed adolescents. The whole system was 'creaking' and 'sick', she said. Sarah wanted closer communication with mental health services and a community psychiatric nurse in the Practice team. Mental health services were fragmented, not the least because, as she put it, of the size of workloads, while there was little effective liaison between the Practice and the community psychiatric team. People were too busy for that. Provision and providers were in disarray, whatever policy makers and managers might pretend. Resources were essential to team working, for learning and multi-professional development. Illusions and rhetoric needed to be stripped away.

Pressures at Home

As the research unfolded and our relationship strengthened, Sarah confided in me about difficulties at home and how these exacerbated those at work and vice versa. Private and public roles were blurred in her story, as in most of the narratives. There was a problem with boundaries as patients would often contact her at home. Many were from her ethnic background, as noted in Chapter 5, and it was hard, sometimes, to say no. Moreover, the culture from which she came was intensely patriarchal, and her motherly role clearly prescribed. Her husband, a busy professional, was often absent from the emotional traumas of the family, like many men, she said.

She told me about her young son who was making more demands at a time when work was getting stressful:

... I notice my son used to say to me – oh no, Mum, it is so and so on the phone, please don't go out now. Please, please stay at home and stay with me. So it was obviously also having an impact on my family, my children were starting to be a bit irritated.

... I felt guilty about my work ... I think in every household the woman takes a larger division of the labour at home than the man. Even though my husband helps me a great deal, I think there is always unequal division. It is up to me to organise the shopping, the cooking, the baby-sitting, the nanny, taking the children to the hospital and so on. He will help change the nappies, and do the cooking, if I ask him to, but I think it is unequal ... I don't get a lot of understanding at home. So I am not able to offload anything on my mind on to anybody else. I have to keep it on board and I find that very hard.

... I think it is cultural to a great extent. It is a specific thing that my husband doesn't want to talk about the problems he has at work and doesn't expect to hear my problems and yet I would say to him occasionally when I get a bit angry about it that we don't communicate with each other and I want him to tell me what a lousy day he had at work, if he had a lousy day and he says – why should I offload my problems on to you when we come home? Whereas if he doesn't offload his I can't offload mine and I need occasionally to talk about mine. Perhaps it is just a reflection of our relationship as well, not being as ideal as it could be.

Sarah was trying not to overdo things:

I was feeling very tired ... I took a break. All my friends thought that it was revolutionary to go off on your own ... It was having a break away, not only from the Practice, but also my family, because I have a two-year-old daughter and a seven-year-old son, who make demands on my time physically and mentally. Lots of homework to do every night and my daughter is at an age where I have to pick her up a lot, because she needs her nappy changing still and she is very clingy to me when I am around. Perhaps because she doesn't see a lot of me. So it is really having a proper break away from the family responsibilities, cooking, cleaning, looking after the children and a break from the Practice ... I try to involve my family with the Practice, although I am saying, I am contradicting myself in a way because I said I try to leave it behind when I go home, but I want my family to see my work as being part of their life. I don't want them to resent it, or feel that it is something that they are not, that they are excluded from. So my son, I sometimes bring him down to the surgery ... Yes he is seven and he will sit behind reception or he will sit in one of the spare rooms while I am having surgery, and pop in, go out to reception. Talk to the receptionists, talk to the patients, so he will be involved and he loves coming here. He likes it particularly when everybody is here, but I have to limit it to times when the surgery is very quiet because obviously I don't want him to get in the way. Or people to complain about him being here. But I bring him down and he knows all the staff and I think I would like to do that with my daughter when she is a little older as well, so that she feels that it is part of life that they shouldn't resent the Practice taking me away from them.

Her son was not doing very well at school by the time of the third interview a few months later:

I am an inadequate mother and to blame for his poor school performance. But yet I know that that is not the real reason he is not performing well at school. So I try not to let it get to me. I know that he is not performing well at school because perhaps it is just because he is a poor pupil.

... I have always found it difficult to be everything to my patients and everything to my family. It is impossible, but I hope that I have reached some sort of a compromise that leaves them both happy. But I do often feel guilty that my family suffers as a result of my work and I feel that I should be giving them more. And I think my patients are getting as much as I can possibly give them.

Sarah told me that GPs learn to expect little sympathy for how they feel. Many GPs were having a hard time but tended to bottle up their feelings. They were supposed to cope, that is what the myth prescribed. Reality meant self-prescribing tranquillisers. This was Prozac in a colleague's case; he was suffering depression, as Sarah had done. The colleague 'stocks himself on Prozac at the weekend. He is a GP not very far away. And I said "For goodness sake why don't you go to your GP?" and he said "Well I didn't want it to go down on my record, so I prescribed for myself." I was surprised. Shocked.' But it happens all the time, Sarah said.

A Son's Illness

Matters came to a head when her son Daniel was diagnosed as having 'a malabsorption syndrome'. He had to be admitted to hospital, and had a general anaesthetic and an intestinal biopsy. This confirmed the diagnosis and he was put on a gluten-free diet. To have a gluten-free diet, for a seven-year-old, meant giving up bread, pasta, cakes, biscuits, sweets; so many things have gluten in them, she said. Daniel was ill at a time the Practice auditors arrived:

> Over a period of a couple of months he was failing to thrive, vomiting, losing weight, his abdomen distended, like a child with malnutrition. It happened quite suddenly. He became very ill during the first week in August and we cut our holiday short and came back and he was admitted and investigated and now he is on this gluten-free diet, which he has improved dramatically on.
>
> ... Yes, it was hard going, we had the audit committee and he was ill all that time, but we hadn't got a definitive diagnosis until about two weeks afterwards.
>
> ... Well you know I felt very depressed. It is very depressing to be told your child has got a chronic illness. I couldn't give a stuff about the audit committee.
>
> ... Oh yes, people expect you to have made the diagnosis yourself and to know all about it and to know more about it than anybody else, when really you are just another mother to your children, aren't you? You don't look at them as patients. I don't think you look on your family as patients. I didn't notice that he had this problem. I mean I did eventually, but the diagnosis itself didn't strike me down. I was very shocked at the time and I feel that you know GPs do tend to present with all sorts of rare medical problems and it does seem unfair.
>
> Well GPs and their families seem to suffer with lots of rare medical conditions.
>
> ... I mean a GP goes into hospital to have a baby, everybody else has a normal delivery except the GP who ends up having an emergency Caesarean with every complication under the sun. I just think that GPs always seem to suffer from, it is just my observation, lots of rare problems. I am sure statistics won't support it, but you ask other female GPs and they seem to perhaps coincidentally have had a lot more rare problems in their lives than other families. I think we are just unlucky.

Sarah wanted to spend time with her son and felt guilty for not doing so. She wanted to monitor his diet carefully and to make him happy. There was the constant, nagging feeling that she was not giving enough. But when she was working, she asked herself, what could she do? She was caught in the middle of needy worlds. Work was greedy and the Practice had employed management agents who proved to be incompetent and she had to keep a close eye on them. The Practice was in deficit and she felt responsible. She knew, she said, that she had done everything in her power to manage the fund appropriately but some factors were beyond her control, such as the number of hospital referrals.

Daniel's case was being reviewed by the hospital and he was visiting a second consultant, every three months. He needed to take medication daily while his growth rate was kept under constant review.

> So where it is dietary it is also physical as well. It is long term. It does have some long-term physical repercussions if his diet isn't strictly adhered to and he continues to suffer from other features of mal-absorption. But fortunately he seems to be making quite good progress but it is an on-going thing. It is never going to disappear.
>
> ... Certainly when he has days when he is not well, I feel inadequate in assessing him fully because he is my son and I can't look at him objectively. I certainly feel guilty for not spending more time with him. I would like to spend more time. But you feel like you get on a sort of roundabout and you can't get off with work and constant patient demand ... it is very hard to find protected time with your family. And I know that he needs me more than ever, but apart from going part time or retiring early I don't see how I can ever get to spend more time with him because the demands on our time are endless.
>
> You can't shift that responsibility to somebody else ... I don't feel that I could say to my GP you sort this out for me because they will say 'Well you are a doctor aren't you? What do you think?' And instead of them taking full responsibility they won't do that will they? So it is back to me to take some of the responsibility for my family's problems. I mean if my GP didn't know I was a doctor then they would treat us in a different way, but they sort of expect you to take some of the responsibility.
>
> ... I expect that I should be able to help my family and cure them of everything and I certainly do provide them with medication for lots of minor problems at home. But there are times when you really want to offload that burden don't you, on to somebody else. You can't make a decision about your family all the time.

Superwoman was required for this particular script.

A Divided Self

Sarah said she was cutting herself into little pieces. She was 'handing little bits to my family, a lot to my patients and a little bit to the PCG, a little bit to our fund'. She felt torn apart by everybody and distressed that she was not spending sufficient time with her young family. She was angry with some patients for failing to realise that she had a life beyond them and the surgery. She was not coping terribly well, at the moment, she said apologetically. She felt run down, had a cold and sore throat. 'Are other GPs in the study like me?' Sarah asked anxiously. 'Many,' I said. A prime motivation in her life had been to become a good doctor and she wanted to prove herself in a career. Failure was unbearable. But it was hard going just now.

Autobiographical Roots

Sometimes, I could only listen empathically. Sarah talked of caring in the context of her life history. Her parents were first generation immigrants and had struggled, as people from their background did, she said, with running restaurants and trying to establish themselves in a new culture. All their hard-earned money went into privately educating their children. But her youngest brother died of leukaemia. He had been so proud of his older sister. Sarah was about to begin training at medical school when he died and it drove her towards the conviction that she would never let her parents or 'poor brother' down. Her father had died when she was only seven and her stepfather was an unpleasant man, not to be relied on. Sarah learned, early and experientially, to rely on herself, and that there were others who needed her support; she was mother, maybe father too, from an early age. She was still attending a SDL group, but less frequently. Her learning plan was 'on a back burner, just now'.

Recovering Gender

Stories are always contingent, open to revision, and never complete, like the lives they reflect and constitute. Gender, in any explicit sense, was absent from the first interview with Dr Claire Barker, yet it came to occupy a central place in her story. She had been too busy getting through the day and week to give work, home, and 'the norms' which underlay them, much thought, she said. Her two children were there, at the first interview, playing while we talked. Claire made a conscious effort, on her day off, to give the children all the time and attention she could. She wondered why she was talking to me, except she was interested in the topic. She currently worked three and a half days a week but this was often full time when on call. She tried to keep home and work separate but was not always successful. Her husband was a highly successful professional man and they were, at one level, a fortunate family:

... One of the reasons that we both work so hard is that we can earn the money to ... I mean we lived in an area where state schools are extremely good and to be fair I haven't looked around the state schools here but I do know there are bad schools, which means that anybody who has got any money at all sends their child to private school. So we are very pleased both of our children are going to a private school which must be one of the most expensive schools around. And I think that, well, if I am paying for them to have a private education, well paying for them or not, if I am wanting them to do well at school, which I do, I want them to achieve their potential, I think I would be disappointed if, when they are adults, they stayed at home and looked after the kids. Therefore as a role model I think it is quite reasonable to me to go out to work. I talk to them about my work. I don't break any confidentialities, but they have some pluses with my working and there are some downsides.

At that moment Ami and Tim wanted their mummy and the tape was switched off. Mummy and I tried to explain what the research was for, but a little hand tugged her away from the interview. There were other, more pressing priorities.

A Husband and a Changing Story

The arrangement with her husband was reasonable, she insisted. They often discussed sharing responsibilities and were lucky to have sufficient income to employ a nanny four days a week (the nanny was on holiday that day). There was a cleaning lady, too, who came once a week. Claire and her husband made sure they had time for themselves. She went to a gym to keep fit. She was a fortunate woman indeed, compared to many patients. She was engaged in a number of learning projects, which included group skills training in a voluntary organisation.

The story changed three months later. She had thought about the issues raised in the previous interview. She was happy afterwards, she said, but her main thought had been about 'a very rosy view of being a female GP and having a family and it isn't as easy as I made out on that occasion'. The transcript had captured most of what she felt at the time but the issue she really wanted to address was the conflict between being a female doctor and a mother at the same time:

> ... I think that almost a week later it was the classic example that despite having all this wonderful childcare, and help in the house, my husband was supposed to be home at a certain time, because I had some work commitment. In fact I had to work for the GPs' cooperative, the out of hours cooperative and he wasn't home and that brought it home to me that now that I am at a new surgery ... and it is that big difference

that really at the end of the day he doesn't have to worry. All he has to worry about is his job. He doesn't have to worry, although he is very good and we have talked about it, he doesn't have to worry about the home issues. Whereas for me when I am on call it isn't just the stress of being on call, in fact that is the least stress, it is making sure the children, are they dressed for school, have they got their things in a satchel, has the nanny turned up on time? How do I balance all those things? And in fact I got quite angry with him a week afterwards, probably because of saying all those things and saying 'yes it is all fine' and then I felt totally let down because he wasn't there and I had to do some juggling act, and I was late for the cooperative which I don't like being.

... We have talked about it, he makes no bones about it that he cannot take on what I did. He cannot take on the responsibility for the running of the home, overseeing the nanny, being responsible for the children. What he can manage is his job and he works very hard, which obviously does benefit both of us, but he can't take on those other responsibilities. He doesn't feel able to. He said to me – I cannot guarantee actually that I will be there at any time on a given evening because if something does arise then I am going to deal with it. So for instance I am normally on call on a Tuesday here. I have now employed my nanny to stay until 7.30 on the understanding that if I get a visit or a section I am not going to be home till later. I am going to phone her up and ask her to stay on, whereas my husband never actually has that worry because either my nanny or I am at home. There is the ultimate responsibility of who actually looks after the children.

A parents' evening brought matters to a head:

... normally when I go along to parents' evening everything is absolutely fine, my nearly four-year-old has just started at nursery and I went along expecting to hear everything was absolutely fine. In fact they said 'Well we think he has some speech problems', which I have noticed myself and I had raised at a previous nursery and I had had his hearing checked in case he had a hearing problem. They were quite concerned and I said 'Well I will organise another hearing test and I am quite happy for him to have speech therapy', but I came away from that with the emotions of obviously it is very upsetting. You never want to hear there is anything wrong with your child. It is not a major thing and I think with speech therapy it will be corrected, but I also came back feeling terribly guilty for working as hard as I do. And in fact I know rationally that it would make absolutely no difference if I didn't work and I was at home all day. He has got an excellent nanny who has got very good pronunciation, enunciation, a wide vocabulary. His elder sister has no language problems at all, although she did have because she has had two sets of grommets and has had hearing problems, but I think that is one of the gender issues and I obviously spoke to my husband and he said – 'Don't be so silly, nothing to do with whether you work or not', but I think inevitably as the woman or the mother you come back, or I came back, feeling very guilty and I said 'OK we will organise a hearing test.' I have asked the school to organise speech therapy through the school, because I feel that would be less traumatic for him if he is taken out of his nursery for an afternoon in a school environment. And I was thinking, well I will take some time off work to go along to that, but of course these things are very difficult to manage. I have taken my holiday to go on my course I am doing. I have got two courses up until Christmas. I have taken all my holiday, so I am going to have to go along to my partners, when it arises, and say 'Look, I would like to be able to take this time, please will you let me take it?' ... And that is one thing that my husband isn't going to have to do. I mean I want to do it and I am sure, to be fair to him, that he would like to do it, but he wouldn't feel the same need, the same drive, to try and be there for him, for that.

The gendered edge of a 'fortunate woman'; Claire said it was not so much receiving the transcript that had the impact, rather reflecting on the interview. She told her husband how she felt, and, as it happened, our interview was taking place just after their discussion. Had I seen her another day, in another week, it might have been a different story, she said. She was finding it hard to be a good and empathic GP when she was so worried about her son and sorting out his problems.

Gender and Style as a Doctor

We were to talk a great deal about gender in the role of the doctor, as well as in learning, over the course of the research:

> ... I will come over as much more slanting towards the feminine side and I think I am seen as being more empathic, more in touch with my emotions, more willing to talk about them... You can't say that all women are going to be in touch because here, for instance, there is someone, a man, who is very empathic.
> ... I think because I have done a lot of, recently, group work and then we have been given feedback and talked about things. I think that is

sort of the way I have been seen by the people. It is certainly something I aim to be. I see myself as facilitating the consultation, not running the consultation ... I am quite happy to talk about sexual issues with patients. I am quite happy to talk about depression. I am quite happy to talk about the ins and outs of people killing themselves, which, I think, some doctors don't like to do. Equally I am quite happy, if a male patient comes in, I am quite happy to see a male patient. I am quite happy to examine them. They sometimes find it a bit difficult, but it doesn't bother me. I think, I am not a lesbian, but I prefer seeing women. I prefer being with women on the whole. I feel because it is easier to communicate. They are more empathic and they are more honest. Not all, that is a very sweeping statement, but that would be my ... I am quite happy that on the whole I see mostly female patients and children because I feel I can relate well to them.

... I have photographs of my children up in my room, which is something I cautiously thought about for someone who comes into my room with primary infertility. That could be quite a difficult issue to see that I have got my children's pictures up. Equally I do also have a lot of mums coming in who are having problems with their children and I think, I know that they do find it easier to relate to me because I have got young children. OK, I won't have been through all the things that they are going through, but I will have experienced some of those things and I also understand the mother/daughter relationship from first-hand experience. I think because I know that I have been depressed myself, with my depressed patients I think that has enabled me to be much more empathic and more open with them, and as I said to you, discussing suicide and various issues, to actually talk about that with them without them feeling threatened.

There had been a particular patient that morning:

... she came in and I felt she was very much sizing me up, what was I going to be like and she actually came in and said that her husband saw depression as a weakness in your personality. Then she carried on and as the consultation went on it was quite obvious that she was depressed and when we started talking about that I asked her how she felt about depression and actually she sees depression as a weakness. And I feel, and again I discussed this with her, that is why she hadn't actually been able to talk to anyone else. She hadn't been able to talk to her husband, her sister, anybody, friends, about it because she saw it as a weakness. And I think that once she had sized me up and I said to her, I made it quite clear, that I didn't see depression as a weakness, I saw it as an illness just as I saw diabetes as an illness, appendicitis as an illness, I felt that did enable the consultation to go much better and I feel sure she will come back and see me and she was willing to accept help. And again, without breaching confidentiality, she was also a medical person. And it is, I mean this is a very big issue, the issue of stigma related to various illnesses, and it isn't just depression and mental illness, I think there are other illnesses which are stigmatised.

... I actually listened for quite a long time. There were quite a few pauses, which I am sure if I had timed them, weren't long, but I sat through them, which enabled her to keep going. And then I suppose I tried to reflect back to her some of the things that she had said to me and I felt I was very honest with her in the way I was talking. I mean I was relating my own experience, just as if I had diabetes I wouldn't say to a patient – 'Oh yes I have got diabetes and I inject insulin', I wasn't doing that, but was talking to her in a lot of detail about her depression and what she was experiencing. Talking to her about how it felt for her to be depressed rather than just running through, 'Are you sleeping, are you eating, are you tearful? OK fine, are you suicidal? Well here are some tablets.' What did she want to do? And came to a sort of management plan with her. And I actually asked her, I said, 'I would like you to come back and see me. Will you? Do you want to? Would you like to come back?' And she said she would. So I felt that even in the short space of a ten-minute consultation, it was only ten minutes, which is always the thing that amazes me, that we did actually build up a rapport with each other. But I think also she could sense that I really didn't see it as a weakness and that I valued her ...

Claire had taken drugs for her own depression. She had also learned to suffer in silence.

Attracting Some Patients

We talked about men and women patients, including male aggression in the consulting room. We talked about how particular patients insisted on seeing her, and the staff would tend to refer them to her, because she was the GP with a reputation for listening. That morning there was a patient who was suicidal and a nurse had asked if Claire would visit her. A male colleague was available but the nurse and patient wanted her:

I didn't want to see her because it would have wrecked my entire surgery, and it is that dilemma. Do you see the one possibly very needy person and all the other people who have been waiting two and a half to three weeks to see you are then put back an hour and maybe don't see you? And again the visit I did today was someone who had never seen me, she said she only wanted Dr Barker. Well as there was only one visit and I had time to do it, I did it. But I actually felt amazing. I was talking to my partner at lunchtime and said how uncaring can you get as a doctor that someone comes in and begs to see you as they are suicidal and want to see a female doctor and the reply comes back – 'No I am sorry, see the person you should see.' ... I think it is quite onerous being the only female in the practice and I would like another female doctor I suppose.

I don't know about what attracts them. I think that if someone comes in and they are depressed I am highly likely to make the diagnosis rather than saying, rather than sending them away saying they have got a sore throat. I am very open to making a diagnosis just as one of my partners is and I think as I said before when medical students sit in with us they actually make the comment that we see more patients with psychiatric illness than our other two partners. My belief is that because we are probably more open to psychiatric illness, we are more empathic on that particular front and the patients, having seen us once for something, realise that and then are able to see that.

Some doctors in the study talked of 30 per cent of their patients having psychological problems. Claire challenged the figure and said it depends on what you are willing to see and respond to. A sore throat could be the starting point for a bigger story. Many doctors closed their hearts and minds to certain cues. They could not, or did not want to see, the whole picture.

Superwoman

Claire was a diligent doctor who believed in lifelong learning. But it was also a source of division:

I feel very guilty, because I felt I sort of failed, but that is because of the standards I set myself.

... I find it very hard to be a good GP and to be a good mother and to be a good wife, because I set very high standards and I expect myself to reach those standards all the time. And therefore it makes it much easier to fail and I know that is a fault. I mean for instance I hate upsetting anybody. I wouldn't want to upset someone, patient, colleague, husband, child – whatever. I don't like, I always try and consider other people first. I mean I do value myself and I do look after myself but I don't like causing any upset at all. So yes it is very easy for me to end up feeling guilty because I feel I should be there and it does make it difficult. I was saying I didn't see my husband as he didn't get in until eleven and I was in bed by that time ... So I do find it very difficult when it is all the clinical issues of making sure that you are totally up to date and can deal with all those issues, and all the emotional issues. Not letting your patients down or your family. I mean my daughter said to me this morning, 'But Mummy it is parents' assembly. Why aren't you coming?' 'I have got to go to work darling.' ... It is very hard, it is very hard. That is why I go home at the end of the day and I am exhausted. Yes, I could have much easier mornings if I stuck to the old model of the doctor. 'Hello, what is wrong with you? OK fine, here you are, off you go.' I mean I can do that. We can all do that in three minutes. One of the things that I changed when I came here was that I said I have got to have ten minutes for every consultation, whatever it is, however small. Even the extra is fine. I will just do longer surgeries, which is actually what I do. I do longer surgeries.

Claire Barker wanted to be a good doctor, wife and mother. She was throwing herself into her training but felt anxious a lot of the time. Feelings of depression were never far away, and a child's illness loomed. If she was managing this patchwork existence it was at a price; in a gendered world where men, at work and home, were too often emotionally absent and yet emotionally demanding most of the time.

Changing Places

Gender featured prominently in Jane Kelly's story, in relation to patients and in her own intimate relationships:

A patient started off only bringing in physical symptoms, and wanting a physical diagnosis and then managing to get her to accept that actually this was all stress-related. But still you have always got this difficulty that they present as one person without the rest of the family and it is only in time that you actually find what is going on in the family. Time eventually revealed that her new partner, who she has now married, is out of work, long-term unemployed and I think there was some health-related thing. Not that he was terribly ill but just could not do this particular job, bad back or something, and she has got – I am not sure whether it is two or three children from a previous marriage and then they have got a baby together. Once she had accepted that it was depression, she then made it into post-natal depression because that was more acceptable, but then that didn't seem quite the picture and eventually it came out that her daughter by the previous marriage has got attention deficit disorder and so is actually a quite difficult child to parent. The new partner can't cope with her and although he is at home and should be helping her and helping with the baby, because he has got time to do things, he was absenting himself from the family situation and if he was around just rowing with the daughter. So actually what was going on really needed some family therapy and sorting the parenting issues out, and stepfather/stepchild issues and unemployment issues and financial stresses. That takes time to tease out and in general practice you haven't got a lot of time to do that. And once you have teased it out then what do you do about it? You can't do the family therapy yourself because you haven't got time to do it and there isn't any family therapy available in this area, so you are a bit stuck.

... when you look at the type of patients that come to the female doctors and the issues they bring, they do bring much more emotional stuff that they wouldn't necessarily bring to the male partners. Although that varies because obviously you get a male partner who perhaps has a bit of the feminine gender thing so that people will be similarly open and share the emotional stuff. The patients do select which doctor to see in a group practice by which problem they have got. You know that some of the people that come to see me regularly will happily see one of the male partners with a sore throat or cough or cold sort of thing but if they actually want to continue discussing their ongoing issues then they wait to come and see me again ... I think they can perceive quite quickly who would listen and who would respond in the way that they want. They don't want someone to just say – 'Oh pull yourself together.' And so they have worked out that you are the sort of person who would be empathic and sympathetic maybe, whatever the need is. Then they do that. It is this calling card business isn't it? They will come and check you out with something fairly ordinary and then in the first consultation or a subsequent one bring the real issue. Patients do discern who is going to deal with them ... My male partners are split really. One of them does and has equally long and difficult consultations as the female partners and the other two are much more matter of fact and clinical and run on time.

There was a conspiracy, at times, in general practice, Jane said. Many male patients preferred drugs and a quick fix to talking cures. Some male doctors squirmed at the thought of emotional engagement with their patients. Drugs were a quick and easy fix for them too.

An Activist

Jane Kelly was also one of only two female doctors on the local PCG:

I think from the outset I was intrigued by the vision of joint working across health, social services, all the different team members of primary care. To actually look strategically at what was going on and to try and address local needs. So from the beginning my interest was on the wider picture as opposed to, for me, as an individual. And I think I just felt very strongly ... that was the way forward for health. There was no way that the health budget was going to be able to cope with all the stuff that were really social issues or whatever, and unless we actually worked together we were never going to cope. And I suppose I didn't really want other doctors that I didn't feel had the same views as myself being the ones to run the thing. That is probably what it is and the fact that you know there is a danger that it could become very money-orientated, worrying just about the individual GP and where they fit in the picture and not actually looking at the population of the area and what we can do to better their health.

... Well I think that the person who ever thought of the idea was actually probably trying to take away the hierarchical role and the absolute sort of GP is the be-all and end-all and everyone is subservient to him. I think that is what they are trying to do away with. And so I think what they are wanting is that we have to accept that we are part of a team delivering primary health care services and appropriately referring on to secondary and tertiary services with the ultimate aim to better the health of the patient, but also spend the least amount of money. And I think that we have got to recognise that we are not the be-all and end-all and there are many other professionals within primary care that are better at certain jobs than we are and being prepared to send the patient in the right direction really. But I don't think many doctors like that, because it is not the way they work. I am the only woman GP at any of these meetings apart from one co-opted woman GP on the Board ... So it is male-dominated, very much so in this area. This place is very male-dominated.

Jane was wondering about career directions. She questioned being a GP and she was interested in hospices and began to work in one, part time:

And that came out of the blue. I hadn't even really thought about it and got phoned up by one of the retired consultant paediatricians locally to say they needed doctors to work there ... but she obviously knew me from referrals and things. Was I interested? So it is bringing together an interest in paediatrics and the hospice and what I wanted to do, but children's hospice work is very different. All the children's hospices in the country are staffed by GPs in fact. So it is ten years behind the adult hospice world, so it is taking on GPs, so I am pursuing my specialist interest.

... Because children's hospices are mainly respite care rather than fully terminal care, they don't have the need for full-time doctors, but they do have the need for full-time doctor cover and I don't know why, I don't understand why, but they have really struggled to find any doctors prepared to do it. Whether the timing is bad with the Primary Care Groups, or whether we are all just overworked I don't know. So when they first asked me I sort of said 'I can't really fit it in with what I am doing' and I really oscillated around a bit. I really wanted to do it because it is an area where I could see my skills being well used but couldn't see how it could fit in ...

She liked listening to people and their stories:

So I suppose that has a fascination for me for people and the time and opportunity to draw that out of people and to facilitate the process that they are going through when they know they are dying. I find that, what is the word, not a blessing, but it is just very rewarding that people involve you in that process and I think I am not a generalist, which is why I have found general practice very difficult. And the hospice skills, it is quite a defined area, quite easy to become skilled very quickly in pain control, once you have learnt it, you get quite skilled at it, symptom control, and so there is a great reward and pleasure in helping someone die well. I think when you are in acute hospitals and you see the bad deaths, that is distressing, whereas if you are in the hospice to be able to facilitate a good death for people, and the relatives, and so on is just so rewarding. And I suppose death is inevitable, so to actually make death a better process is rewarding. I suppose I find that side of it rewarding and I suppose my faith doesn't make it quite so hard to live with death as it might do.

I think the opportunity for the person to explore some of the things that are the unfinished business is good. And I think the opportunity to relieve the suffering, that is always appreciated by the patient. They will often say when they first come, 'the great fear of dying of cancer is the pain', and when you can say 'you know we can control your pain and you must let us know and we will do what we can', that is very rewarding. And it is very rewarding to see the relief to the relatives because their fear of death is often the pain and the symptoms, and so that I think makes a good death when you can see that the relatives are peaceful with the way that the person is dying. So it is a combination of physically sorting out the symptoms, but also emotionally and spiritually sorting out, helping them to make sure they have sorted things. I think one of the things about dying of cancer is that you have got time, and I always think it is a shame when it is not used. I think sudden death is harder probably to deal with, because of the unfinished business.

... Being able to listen, but also I think you need to be able to quickly process things because they need to know that you have heard and so subsequent questions are relevant to what they have said, which I think some doctors are good at quickly processing, but they don't then give the patient a chance to speak, so they don't have the listening side, and I think some listeners are very good but they don't process quickly enough. So often they then make inappropriate replies and the person thinks 'Well actually they didn't hear what I was saying because they have got that wrong.' So I think you have to have both really in that sort of sphere. The listening I am doing is not like counselling because I am not just letting them work it out for themselves because I am still taking a doctor advisory directive sort of role, but having spent more time getting there, possibly that is the difference. Does that make sense?

... I am often told by my patients in general practice that – 'you are good, you do listen' ... I don't think many doctors in the Health Service have listening skills.

Listening, and knowing when to act, were at the heart of the work.

Doubts About Being a GP

Jane was increasingly unsure about being a GP. She had originally planned to be a paediatrician but she chose family life instead. She had found the research useful, she said, towards the end, in reconsidering options and in mapping the important influences in her biography:

In general practice you do get continuity with your patients ultimately, but in ten-minute bite-sized chunks not in an hour-long meeting ...

I was amazed at the diversity of HIV work. I thought it would be homosexuals or drug addicts and they weren't at all, actually ... I think probably between the two sessions there have been ten people. I think two, no three, were homosexuals I think, out of the ten I saw. One was a girl from Africa who acquired it in Africa. One was a Scottish girl who I think had probably acquired hers from, oh no that's right she, I don't know if you have heard the story, but there was a sex ring on a local estate, wife swapping-type thing some years back and most of them are infected. I think she was part of that. There was a chap who got it from blood, a donation, and then there was a newly diagnosed couple that the girl, we don't know where they got it, but we presume that the girl got it from a previous boyfriend who was a drug addict and then she got married to a South African chap and she has passed it on to him. So you know there is a cross-section of people, it is fascinating. I just find it … I think I like it because I find people fascinating rather than anything else. So it wasn't as I expected it to be at all really. I really expected a much narrower group of the population, but I suppose with most of them to some extent it picks certain groups – it does actually affect a cross-section of the community.

Her son's illness, and her own, focused her mind, and that of her partner:

… we have actually had to face the possibility of death and so it is not unfinished for us, if you see what I mean. I had – it wasn't imminent – but I had a carcinoma in situ of the cervix and I could have, it could have progressively recurred. I had to have two operations and a hys-terectomy and so because we communicate well, we talked, even at that stage about the possibility, so I suppose because we have explored it as a couple, it is not particularly such a problem and I have had a mis-carriage, so we have had that loss to deal with as well. And then our son had picked up an abnormality when I was pregnant and they debated whether he had Downs and all sorts of stuff, so we had a very traumatic pregnancy and then he had to have a fairly major operation when he was born, so we have been through some of those things as well. So we have had our own stresses and because we communicate well, and because of our faith I think, and supports we have had from friends and family, we have been through that. So I think I am probably fortunate to be fairly secure and know where I am that these things don't perhaps quiver me quite as much. Sometimes they do. I have to say my husband has probably been the biggest security in that I know if I mess up on something I do at work, or in one of these presenta-tions, or something like that, he still loves me. It is not going to alter what he feels about me. So his love is unconditional, so I don't have to actually prove myself to him. I think that has made an enormous difference.

Changing Spaces

Jane shared the transcripts with Tom, her husband. He had gone through bad times at work and was now training as a therapist:

> and then we had a sudden revelation the other week, that I could actually work full time, so I could do half time hospice and stay with my half time in the practice and my husband could stop working so that he could pursue his interest, because he is doing a diploma at the moment and everyone keeps telling him that the second year of the diploma is very hard work and he will never fit it in with what he was doing, and because doctors obviously earn more, my half time should hopefully come to his equivalent of his full time. So that is what we decided to do. A week ago.
>
> It was like a step of faith really, because we haven't had it all confirmed yet. I have got a formal interview with the hospice next week and I don't know quite how much they are going to pay me and I want to keep some Primary Care Group involvement going. I don't know how much that will generate in terms of pay, but I am hoping I can juggle it around, and knowing that my husband will be home for the children, I am happy to do that. I wouldn't work full time and use childcare, paid childcare, with him looking after them.
>
> I suppose Tom and I tend to talk a lot about our days and what has been happening, not dumping, but in a sort of structured sense. We always make sure at some point in the day we both talk through what we have been up to, so if there has been any particular burning issue I usually will talk it through with him. And I miss it when I don't. So we quite often end up going to bed very late if one of us has been out at a meeting and it is sort of half ten or eleven before we even start having that offloading, but we always do, and I think we both need that. So that is probably where most of it goes, which I don't know, some people have sort of confidentiality boundary problems don't they, but Tom is better on the confidentiality than I am I think, so I don't have any problems there. As to when you have had a bad day and the rest of the family are bearing the brunt of it, this is inevitable whatever job you are in really, and I am aware that sometimes I know if I am feeling really tense and have got less patience with the children, but I don't think they suffer too badly.

Tom was changing too:

> Well I suppose because my husband is now a househusband we have much more of a partnership in family life than many couples. In fact Tom is probably more maternal than I am. He worries more about some of the things about the children and their safety and where they are at more than I do. So I think in our particular relationship we don't have that issue, but I am sure if I had married somebody else I could have quite sympathised with that issue. That, as you say, not only are you expected to do all the work, but also to do all the work when you get home as well. So I think that is very fortunate with Tom really. And also he's ... back to gender, he has got a lot more feminine in him than many men and therefore is much more in tune ... he is much more into that sort of thing and thinking about people's reactions and emotions and is much more sensitive to things. Usually he reminds me to ring and see how my mum is and says – 'Oh your mum didn't look that well' – and I hadn't really noticed you know.
>
> ... One of the study things I went on years back about HIV was looking at sexuality, because obviously at the time it was mainly the homosexuals who were infected, and they were talking about the mixture in all of us of the male and the female and that we are all, you know some are on a mixed spectrum and there isn't this clearly defined male and female. I find that concept very helpful and also in practice you know I have seen it to be very true, and I think that society hasn't taken that on board and that a lot of the difficulties that people get into are because they are not allowing the other part of them to surface. And I think that relationships is often an issue isn't it, in work, and not knowing why you are reacting or feeling that if a man is reacting in what is perceived to be a feminine way then there is something wrong with him. And I think we need to educate society that there is a spectrum and a mix and I think possibly why Tom and I balance each other quite well is actually he is a man with a lot of feminine in him, and I am possibly a woman with a lot of masculine in me. And I think that we probably balance each other very well for that reason. And I think that he would have done very badly in a relationship with a very feminine woman because of their demands on him; he perhaps wouldn't have been comfortable with that. You know you get these sort of weak women who expect the man to make all the decisions, whereas I think because we are both a mix, in different situations, you know I expect him to take the decision making, but in other situations I will get on and do it.

Society was grappling, she said, with gender, at every level, as were individual people in particular lives:

> And it works very well for us and you know we just seem quite comfortable with the way it is working out. Interestingly the children still want Mummy for a lot of the emotional type of things which I think Tom finds quite difficult because he is, as I said before, he is probably much more the maternal one of the two of us.
>
> Yes I think because he is doing his therapy course he has got a role as a student and so because he is seeing clients and therefore does have a job if you like, although it is not paid, I don't think that has been an issue. I think first time round when we did it when he gave up work completely and he had no job, again he is a very sociable person, so he was going to mother and toddler groups and socialising with the women and enjoying that and accepting that he was being like the mums who had an equally valid role as a parent and their job at that time was the children and he took that on ... I think he is unusual in that ... and then it came up again today talking to someone about teenage pregnancies and sex education in schools and how you can educate as much as you like but actually it is a cultural understanding and how there is this sort of big expectation in society that men and women are vastly different and that they don't overlap and that the men are very ... Yes I suppose society has allowed that ... I suppose it is not a problem because we are quite comfortable with it because we are both quite comfortable with being able to be a mix because we have both thought about it. I suspect it wouldn't make for a comfortable relationship if one of you was keen on the idea and the other wasn't. So I suppose for us I just see it as allowing each other the opportunities to do what we are good at and fit comfortably with.

Doing justice to one's own and another's complexity seems to involve what Andrew Samuels (1993) has termed 'psychological pluralism', the capacity to be one person and many in a dynamic and creative interplay. And that involves loving and reciprocal relationships as a basis for sustaining the ontological project of the self. Stephen Frosh (1991) has argued that socio-cultural transformations are mirrored in the internal world, requiring dependable relationships and good objects in order to exploit rather than being overwhelmed by change. Jane and Tom had a secure, dependable relationship which meant, in their case, acknowledging that gender and role need not be socially prescribed, but can be open to constant negotiation. It seems that doing justice to the complexity of one's self, as much as to others, lies at the heart of being the good doctor and a lifelong learner, in a psychological sense. The instability of subject positions, as Frosh (1994) insists, is to be welcomed in these terms, rather than regretted, because escape is possible, however frightening, from the rigid norms of the past.

8
Men Behaving Sadly

If way to the better there be, it exacts a full look at the worst.
Thomas Hardy, 'De Profundis'

A Crisis and New Possibilities?

Feminism, in particular, has taught that human beings invent knowledge with only limited access to potential explanations and limited claims to infallibility. Knowledge is always and inevitably filtered through the gaze of a culture and its power-laden and gendered processes. While everyone, in theory, is free to generate explanations of how the world functions and to devise schemata for organising the objects and events of the world, not all of these will be considered legitimate or are easily articulated. There is selection at work. Those who have power to validate their own models of the world, and themselves, tend to validate their own power in the process (Spender, 1981).

Feminism has also taught that it was particular men who constructed the stories considered most legitimate and 'normal' within our culture, while women, and their experiences, as well as the diverse experiences of many men, tended to be constructed as 'other'. Knowledge, in the academy, for instance, has reflected what powerful men most deified. Seidler (1994) has written of the continuing tendency for men to see reason as the prime source of individuality, and thus freedom and capacity for self-determination. Women, and 'inadequate' men, are supposedly more tied to their feelings, making it difficult for them to act and know decisively. Everyday speech is riddled with gendered assumptions: women suffer emotional outbursts and must learn to calm down and behave rationally, 'like good men should' (Seidler, 1994). There is a profound loss in the schism between thought and feeling, head and heart, and men and women are both the poorer for it. For some middle-aged, male GPs, in a context of a changing role and culture, the disjunction between what is, and what they believe ought to be, can be traumatic.

Bennet (1998), a psychiatrist, has described how reality often disappoints doctors, who become tired and disillusioned with themselves and the health-care system. There may be a plateau in middle life where the loss of further opportunities is interpreted as failure. Doctors must learn to acknowledge their own fallibility, accept their wounds and help from colleagues. They must escape the omnipotent myth of 'needing to know' and of coping in splendid, emotional isolation. This is in part a profoundly 'male' story, to which reason alone has no answer. Understanding feelings, as a medic and a man, is a prerequisite of a more contented life.

Times may be changing, and, as Andrew Samuels (1993) has observed, there is a slow dislodgment of the literal and metaphoric place that 'masculinity' has enjoyed, as the 'subject' and initial premise of most conversations, in medicine and more widely. But many, especially middle-aged male doctors, still struggle in a world where they were taught to be rational and cope. There are two such stories at the heart of this chapter. A third narrative, which concludes the chapter, can be read differently, as a pessimistic perception of the possibilities for a psychologically literate profession, in contemporary times.

The Disturbance of a Man

Ken Ross works in Brent. There are many impoverished and single-parent families in his patch, and a large number of unemployed men without role and apparent purpose. Some men, as well as many women, as Ken put it, drift in and out of prison. Drugs and prostitution are mainstream industries. When we first met, Ken openly admitted to feeling uncertain about himself as a GP and whether he wanted to continue as a doctor. He heard about the research and contacted me, in fact, because of wanting to develop his writing. He felt deeply unfulfilled and was looking for some way out. As it transpired, he misunderstood the project's purpose, but wanted, nonetheless, to continue. His favourite writer was Thomas Hardy, whom he frequently mentioned. He had taught Hardy's work as a schoolteacher, and recalled his struggles with black students who resented the idea of 'black' signifying negative and menacing stereotypes. Some of the themes that obsessed Hardy – the inner conflict between hope and fear, love and despair, and of how the past might stalk the present, and disable the future – haunted Ken too. He was almost fifty.

A Few Regrets

It took some time for the two of us to get to know each other and for him to feel confident in the research. Yet he was also anxious to talk, which underlay his desire to write. He was taking stock and thought writing might help in the search for meaning and new direction. He had recently had an article published in 'one of the freebie GP journals' and wanted to write more, and better. He longed to write a novel but it had to be good because it would be pointless to produce anything else, 'but I don't know how good it will be'. He described spending 'too much time looking backwards, so in that sense taking stock is not a new thing for me and I am often a person who looks back with regret. I know it is wrong, but I still find myself doing it ...'

Medicine and Religion

His religious beliefs were important, and he wondered about God's will for him. He had thought, on many occasions, of becoming a minister in the church. He had also considered, at medical school, being a child psychiatrist. He liked psychiatry and it was the main reason why he wanted to be a doctor. But the comments of particular teachers, and its uncertain, often derided status in the profession, put him off the idea. One surgeon dismissed 'psychiatry' with the remark that 'psychiatrists use a lot of long words, about very little'. It was where 'second raters' ended up.

Paediatrics was another possibility, as was general surgery. However, he lacked confidence in himself as a surgeon, although he tried it for a while. He turned to ophthalmology and had two attempts at the exam, but failed both times. And yet he had sufficient experience of both surgery and ophthalmology to work overseas, in a developing country. He found mission and purpose, for a while. But he never ever felt good enough, and there were some experiences which caused him continuing concern.

'A Mental Problem'

He introduced what he called his 'mental problem' in the first interview and talked about it, at length, subsequently, as he felt more secure in our relationship. He had wanted to train as a counsellor:

> ... I had a mental problem ... after a number of false starts, they did eventually allow me onto the course ... we then spent four months on the course, at the end of which ... I wasn't actually turned down, but deferred in their words, to see if the problem would get better. But I could see the problem continuing so that was a very, very emotional time for me when I was turned down.
>
> ... Yes, I don't know where it comes from or where in a sense it started. It is an obsessional-type problem that I have ... It is not as strong as it

was but it has not gone completely certainly. It is connected I am sure with my tendency to look back and to regret moves that I have made and I know that there were traces of it, looking back, you can remember little incidents. I can remember as a child we owed the milkman ... an old halfpenny and I can remember walking down the road to the shop where the milkman was and saying 'Oh we owe you this halfpenny', and the lady in the shop saying 'How silly of you to come with that, just such a small amount.' And I remember marking a book in the university library and going to the desk to show the librarian I had upset ink on this and she thought 'This is trivial. Why have you brought it?' Things like that that one thinks are connected.... when I was doing a casualty job and found myself checking over things I had done, or thought I hadn't done and so on, with patients and then checking to see if I had dropped a piece of paper.

Ken wondered, self-deprecatingly, if I, Linden, was really interested in his life; in a man of muddled ideas and uncertain purpose. 'Is this what you want for your research?' he asked. 'I am not a clear thinker ... I sit there wondering – "am I wasting this chap's time as well?", some of the things. Because when I feel you have asked a question and I haven't answered it I think 'Oh gosh, what a thickie I am."'

Managing Emotions

He was good with particular patients, he remarked, but by no means all. There was someone who had been to see him that day, just before I arrived for the third interview. The patient suffered chronic anxiety problems, attends regularly and enjoys 'coming to see me and says that he always feels better after he has been with me'. Ken, however, felt differently:

I have to admit that I don't feel better after that person has been here, but that person is able to sound off all his feelings during the ten or eleven minutes he is in here and OK I realise that just him coming to me has been therapeutic. Now anybody could do it. It wouldn't have to be a GP in that role. It could be anybody who befriends this particular patient or gives this person room to express themselves ... Yes. I suppose one does feel it is impossible ... It is the patients that one feels one cannot do anything for and if you have two or three of those in a row ... because each one is heavy, whereas if you have a heavy patient followed by something else, a sore throat or something, it gives you that recovery time. Sometimes, I suppose it can feel a bit like being a dart board sitting here, that you have got a patient throwing darts at you, bombarding you with information. You have heard it all before and you feel this patient hasn't changed and isn't likely to change, but they sound off all these things for ten minutes, often more, and you feel weary at the end of it. I am very, very tired at the end of it and because I am tired I am therefore feeling depressed and it is at that point that one says, 'Is this really what I want to be doing?' So it is purely the fatigue, mental and physical fatigue and going back to mid-life crisis I realise that at fifty I can't take it in the same way I could twenty years ago ... One day runs into another, but ... there was one day last week and it could have been that day, when I was the only doctor here all day. There was a nurse and nurse practitioner and although there weren't hundreds of patients, there were enough patients for me to feel that I had been working hard without a break until 6 or 7 o'clock. I drive up the hill and it is as much as I can do to remember to stop at the red lights and move off on the green ones.

More Guilt, More Hardy

Ken said he majored on guilt:

So I am often very bad at handling my own emotions, but I, I don't know how this sounds, but I am comfortable with someone who is weeping or very sad or whatever. I sometimes sense that there is almost a feeling of guilt that I am too comfortable and enjoying the power that my occupation gives me to be so close, not only so close to someone's emotions, but to sort of give them the room to express their emotions and you can feel that there is a sense of power there that I have got that I can almost induce emotions in other people. Sometimes I feel almost guilty about that, although I can see that it is often therapeutic for the person to be able to express those emotions.

... But certainly looking back over my past I can very easily and frequently recover the disasters and remember the disasters, the things that went abysmally wrong, for whatever reason. Whereas the things that went very well and the people who were very appreciative, they blur into the background. So that is another case where I major on the negatives so.

He described a recent sleepless night when reading the fatalism in Hardy:

... I was reading ... Tess of the D'Urbevilles, which of course is full of doom and gloom, but I mean there had been one event in the past where she had been raped really and that led to other misfortunes ... and I am sure our past does, well, past influences one's present self-view, very much ... my confidence in performing this task is affected by previous exposure to similar tasks in the past and I can also see that, say, if you have an optimistic view of the future then yes it does give you a brighter view of now ...

Over time, he talked more about his past:

... I make mistakes and sometimes, occasionally a bad mistake and then you know that engenders bad feelings in me. But generally I feel I do my job well so I am not threatened by the idea that somebody might want to reassess my performance. In fact I would almost welcome that. But it intrudes on me in the sense that they are going back to the disasters from the past. I think of something that I have done in the past and I think, 'Gosh! what I did then was just as bad as what that chap has done now' and it is appearing on the front page of the *Daily Mail* or whatever it is. So it is back to the word guilt again, isn't it? That comes in because I think I should have been hauled up before the GMC about that, but I wasn't you know. So that intrudes in that way ... It is difficult for me to talk about. I was happy in surgery and other things, it was just that my confidence got severely dented ... I went overseas to stand in for a doctor who was on sick leave and a year became two years and two years became longer, and that was where some of the disasters occurred. But during that time I felt 'Well, I have got all this knowledge in surgery and other things, isn't there something I should be using rather than losing?' ... And the problem that I was encountering repeatedly was that, particularly with surgery which was the commonest thing, I was getting a particular complication with some of the fluid which was coming out of the eye that wasn't meant to come out of the eye, and this happened. Sometimes it was as much as 50 per cent whereas the percentage of that complication should have been perhaps 5 per cent at the most and this was, I attributed, because I didn't have the instruments that I was used to using in England. And so I tried my best with the instruments that I had there and tried to get hold of instruments that were similar to what I had used, but never had access to the same facilities that I had had in this country. Other surgeons managed it, could manage to get really good results, you should see some of the methods, but I couldn't and I got increasingly frustrated with this and nobody was telling me that I had to stop.

... But it was interesting, things like the Bristol heart case where they were getting bad records and the question has been put that why didn't someone blow the whistle earlier? Well there was no one there to blow the whistle on me, but in the end I, in a sense, blew the whistle myself saying, 'I can't stand this, I am getting too depressed at all these complications.' Yes, people were going away seeing that couldn't see before, but the long-term implications of that complication were that they have gone on, a high percentage of them, quite probably, although I didn't see it, probably went on to develop retinal detachment at some stage. So they would have had their vision for some years, but then lost it and I just wasn't happy with that ... And I suspect there are tensions that we haven't, deeper tensions even, that we haven't got to.

The Final Interview

At the beginning of each interview, as I have explained, we spent time identifying themes from the previous session. Ken wanted to talk some more about his low self-esteem and of never being quite good enough. He had recently been appointed a trainer in general practice and was asked, at interview, about problems he might foresee in having a registrar in the practice. He answered the wrong question. The question he answered was about any weaknesses he had. He remembered when being interviewed for a registrar's post, years before, that a member of the panel came up to him after the interview and said it wasn't meant to be self-destructive: 'I had sort of destroyed myself as it were.' Ken asked himself, often, where this destructive voice came from and why he was this way.

He talked about his family of origin. 'Mother could sometimes be negative', but he was unsure of the significance of this. She once made a remark, after a school Speech Day, and it still hurt. He was walking up the road with her and she said how nice it would have been if he had got a prize, like his cousin and another boy. 'Maybe remarks like that could have tainted my whole life', Ken mused.

His father had been a distant and emotionally unavailable figure:

... I can remember when I decided to change from doing English to medicine at the very last minute and Dad again being out of his depth ... but he didn't know what to say in that situation.

... No, but he was older. My mother said to me ... after he died, 'You didn't really have a father, you had a grandfather' because he was forty-nine I think when I was born, an older man. So as I got to the end of my schooling he had reached sixty-five and was retiring ...

There was a book he had read with the title *To Be the Best that I Can Be*. He always had to be the very best, to do more, and reach higher. He was beginning to realise that it set him up for failure and disillusionment. He was driven to be the very best of doctors and could not tolerate failure. His parents were good people, Ken added, but of their time and place. His own children sometimes complained of his unavailability and of being too busy for them. This might be a pattern repeated across the generations and it troubled him.

In the last interview he returned to feeling haunted. He felt responsible for his actions, and that some people would have been better served by a better doctor. There were no other doctors available, in that country at that time, so he knew, rationally, that was an illusion:

> ... The reason those haunt is that every so often one is reminded of them. You read something, there was that midwife recently, a couple of weeks ago, that was hauled up to the Royal College of Midwives and was publicly rebuked because she delivered a child and the child had died ... I can think of very close parallels to that one and I think I said 'there but for the grace of God go I' because I have made mistakes but haven't been, up to this point, haven't been hauled before the General Medical Council. Now those haunt me ... I could have gone into politics. I don't think I would have been very good. But now, knowing that I have these skeletons in the cupboard, which I know about but not many other people know about, I would be very anxious about the thought of offering myself as a potential candidate for a political party because I would be thinking, 'Well what if some reporter, hungry for a story, manages to dig up one of my skeletons and manages to expose this.' In your fantasies you wonder what would you be. I fantasised, the last thing I would want to be would be Minister of Health who would be responsible for the General Medical Council, who at the end of the day might be responsible for counter-signing something which was condemnatory of somebody regarding some misdemeanour they made which was parallel to something I had done. Do you see what I am trying to say? I am not quite so active now, but I do belong to groups which campaign on behalf of people who are tortured or imprisoned or worse in various countries around the world and particularly with the letters you are encouraged to finish with the words: 'I urge you to bring these people to justice.' I hesitate to write those words every time as I think 'Gosh, I haven't been brought to book on some of the things I have done', so these things haunt me.
>
> ... I suppose it is still that desire, that sort of not quite masochistic desire, but that desire to think 'Has justice been done here? Should I have been punished for this? Should I at least have been publicly rebuked for this?' Yes it is still there. I find it difficult to let go of that.

It is these things from the past which were quite devastating where I feel basic mistakes were made, you know, of very gross omissions of care which I regard as wholly indefensible, probably are indefensible one or two of them, then that is not something I like to own up to; that I could have performed so appallingly. And unfortunately for me I could do a hundred things, I could do a hundred things well, but if I do one thing badly I will forget the hundred good things, but the one bad thing will loom large.

'This sound hard', I said. I talked about object relations and how our psyches may be 'peopled' by overly harsh objects, or, in Freudian terms, the overbearing super-ego that plays on fragile self-esteem and could inhibit personal development. All of which led him to a final thought on paths not taken, and possible futures in psychoanalysis:

One often wonders what, how different one would be if one had had the, maybe you have had this, the privilege to have been psycho-analysed ... There was one very interesting time I had and I have often wondered what would have happened. I was a medical student and I had not turned up to a seminar and I felt guilty about this. It was a seminar with a psychoanalyst, child psychiatrist ... I found this man's number in the book and phoned him up to say I am sorry I didn't turn up and there was a little bit of surprise at the end of the phone that I had phoned him up, followed up by – well maybe there are issues here that you would like to discuss – and I backed off, but I have often wondered, what if I hadn't backed off ... because it would have been a very inter-esting time in that I think that time, at the end of medical school, was when some of these mental problems, the obsessional traits and so on, were actually beginning to fix themselves. It was just about then I think that I can identify just one or two incidents. Even that phone call may have been part of that. I have often thought if only I had been brave enough to allow him to work on me at that time. Where would that have taken my life? How different things would have been.

We spent some final moments together considering ways forward. He had a mentor whom he thought might help. He could be someone to talk to, in a profession where it was hard to mention psychological pain and failure. He asked about therapy once more and I shared my experiences and Ken said he would think about it. I thought later about his intense vulnerability. He was driven to be the very best of men, but was unfor-giving when things went wrong. This harsh, inner object world was an impossible burden for any man to bear.

Fathers and Medicine

Dr Ambi Silva's father was ever-present in our four research conversations. He had been an eminent professor of medicine. He was a respected researcher and a hard act for any boy to follow. Ambi was the youngest of eight children, six boys and two girls. There was a big age gap between him and his eldest brother, some twenty years in fact. His brother became a professor in medicine too in a 'very medically biased family'. Ambi was supposed to emulate father and brother. His father was a driven man:

> I can't actually remember ever playing any of the normal childhood activities with my father because his life was medicine, morning, day, weekends and nights. And I was almost brought up to think, so it will be for you too, that is life, but almost a missionary view that this is your mission in life and it was sort of instilled into you. And my father is not alive now, my mother is, but she finds it strange that I am not actively encouraging my children to go into the medical profession. I said that if they wanted it that is fine but I certainly wouldn't be actively encouraging them.

His parents were refugees from the uneasy post-imperial legacy of Empire. They were forced to leave their country because they were unwanted and moved to Britain. Becoming naturalised, in the 1950s, involved being paraded before a man with a bowler hat at Saturday teatime, to be assessed 'as suitably British'. Status, of all kinds, mattered to his parents.

Feeling a Failure

Ambi felt a failure in the eyes of his father. Becoming a GP was 'beyond the pale':

> I was a failure in his eyes ... Oh God, yes, right through to the end of my university time. And then, at university I was fortunate to have a very, very good honours degree, with prizes and so on and I think it was always expected, not just from my parents, but even the sort of people at the medical school. They saw me as someone who was going to end up as a Professor of Medicine attached to the medical school and there was this great surprise, almost a disbelief, when I announced after three years of the post-graduate training that I was going to become a GP.

Ambi got married and a child arrived soon afterwards. He gave up the idea of becoming a professor: there was a family to support and general practice, rather than research, offered an immediate and more substantial income. His father felt let down. He had spent his life ...

'looking down a microscope ... I am sure he had a different view of life and he looked at everything through a microscope.' He couldn't quite understand how anybody could actually do general practice and I think he actually didn't see the purpose of general practice in a funny kind of way. And much to my surprise even my professors in the medical school were very much against it. But things were different at that time. Everybody did go into general practice from my year, most of them, but I suppose they saw me in a different light actually.

His brother was unimpressed too. Ambi was at the bottom of the medical pile and ought to have known better. If this was a private family affair it was one in which culture – surrounding men, status and ethnicity – penetrated to the core.

Justifying Being a GP

Ambi spent much time justifying himself:

A lot of people actually are quite happy if you see them as human beings, they come to you for certain help and you see them as human beings and they see you actually as a fellow human being who hopefully can help them at certain times, and I actually don't think they are necessarily expecting too much of me. But I think ... Gosh, there are all these people there who are quite happy watching Coronation Street; and they talk about that and they really are quite happy watching these things and it gives them not just a superficial happiness, even a sort of inner happiness, and I suddenly realise there are a lot of people out there, yes there is a lot of unhappiness and stress and there are also a lot of people who are quite happy with their lot, as it were. And yet they haven't got much. They may not be professionally trained and anything else and it suddenly made me realise that I need to look at what I am about and what it is that I am trying to do for people. I really don't have to be something I am not.

... I suddenly started realising – hang on a minute – I can actually afford to be who I am. I don't have to try and be someone I am not, because people actually accept it. And I am surprised ... I suppose quite a bit is family upbringing because if you got 98 per cent out of 100 and saying well done, you were told what about that 2 per cent you didn't get. And I think again, within a certain hierarchical medical profession there is that sort of structure anyway. I think within the hospital and particularly the more traditional, the old-fashioned hospital models, it is run that way because it has always been that way and it will always be ... The sort of striving for perfection that actually doesn't have to be, but it is always striving for perfection because this is how it was always done, therefore if it is good enough for me it is good enough for you, because you are another potential consultant in medicine coming up. There is no reason why you can't do it like that ... we were brought up, even within the medical schools, thinking that way, that we were somehow slightly superior beings to everybody else ... my other brother tells me he still feels doctors see themselves as being more superior to him ... And he points out that still we are held in a higher esteem. This is all part of the sort of way people perceived doctors as well.

He often remembered failing to get the extra 2 per cent.

Problems as a GP and as a Person

Learning about people was difficult. He was good at the strictly medical side of the role, such as pharmacology and cardiology. He was good at learning new facts, keeping himself updated:

I need that intellectual stimulation. I cannot have been one of those GPs who for thirty years, sat in the surgery, seeing, which is what it was, sore throats day in day out. They did the thing, went home, came back for evening surgery and that is how it was I am fairly convinced for a lot of people because there were no variations on the theme. It wasn't that and I honestly wouldn't be able to do that. I like a challenge, intellectual stimulation, in things. If it was not for that I think I would get bored with general practice quite easily. Medical things aren't a problem.

It was the 'people side' of the work that bothered him:

Which I am guilty of and it has caused some personal disruption recently, which I have now resolved, but a lot of stress last year. I think I was actually, well I think I needed help last year, put it like that. I didn't seek help because doctors don't. They are supposed to, I dealt with it myself at great pain really last year. It was the latter part of the year. Quite considerable psychological suffering but I don't think people ever knew that really. My own colleagues didn't know about it right till the end when they picked up on it. Perhaps it is not untruthful to say I wasn't far off the edge in my own personal life, but professionally I managed to stay well. If you sat me in front of a psychiatrist you would have said yes I needed to be on a high dose of anti-depressants, but I was perhaps able to hide it. Not at home though – it caused a lot of unhappiness and a lot of pain, it was pain actually, inner pain, which painfully I am beginning to deal with and I think my wife found it very difficult, but we are over the worst, I feel. To me the challenges to general practice are not clinical, not management, that is not the problem ... The difficulty I have is the interaction side of things, that takes more out of me emotionally, psychologically in every sense, more so than this ... I would say I could do that bit standing on my head kind of thing, because it actually isn't a worry, these professional things they talk about. But I think the way we work it is all about interaction, a lot of it is about interaction, a lot about people, what I call 'people management' and people handling and I think you need to start sharing these experiences. Be more clear about where you come from, where other people are ...

He was never trained to handle people and people skills were of low status in the profession.

Anxious for Feedback

Yet Ambi was active and successful as a GP educator. He helped establish, with colleagues, a multi-disciplinary educational group. He was a good facilitator but was always anxious for feedback and reassurance:

But I would be interested to hear how you see some of my experiences manifesting themselves, reflected in what I do with education or any other thoughts of medical interactions, because I suspect a lot of what I have said to you, not only does it affect my doctor/patient life, but I suspect it may have a bearing on me as an educationalist.

... I am aware that you have spoken to other colleagues, general practitioners, admittedly in different circumstances, perhaps from different backgrounds ... and I was sort of wondering whether I am different. Do I have different concerns and problems and different things that I am thinking about compared to my colleagues or am I just the same as the others, because you sometimes wonder if you know your colleagues. You work with them, but you sometimes sort of wonder whether the inner self is perhaps different and we learn in the course of working normally not always to be frank ...

... I do sometimes wonder if there is such a thing as a clone of the average GP. Am I one of those based on my background, the past experiences, am I different? Perhaps we are, by definition, a very varied creature and sometimes I wonder actually whether talking to lots of different GPs you identify certain patterns and perhaps one or two of us are actually different from that.

He wished he could feel more content and not push himself so. The problem went back, in part, to medical school:

So I think there was a little bit of resentment. Perhaps I saw one or two of my sort of fellow students who were with me at that time who pursued that and they were able to kind of do fairly well. I suppose, I probably felt I was more capable at that time and I think it sort of takes you back a bit when you see that and I think I went through a phase of not liking myself. Always sort of feeling I had slightly failed in my sort of pursuits or mission in life. Well I think, I was thirty when I started here at the surgery and I assumed I would work until sixty-five, thirty-eight years in the same place, with the same people. It has its advantages and you see people growing old with you, but if you are also a person who is seeking new frontiers and so on it ... always assumes that you have to be a person who actually isn't going to venture out of your secure environment and more so not wanting to venture. In other words I actually think you have got to be content with your own life and what I call peace with yourself if you were to do that ... I sometimes feel I have given all I have inside me to people and when it comes to my own self I haven't got enough to give myself. I watch all these television programmes about various hospitals and in one of those programmes was actually one of my fellow students who was in my year, and I know that academically I was far more capable, I was always the prize winner and he is the first to admit that he wasn't, and I saw him in relation to some operations. I said to my wife 'the first thing is that his patients are actually quite grateful instantly', I am not saying mine aren't, but you just feel, not unvalued, but you kind of feel – well you know you are battering away at it, battering away at it, but sometimes there is very little to show for it.

Patients go off to hospital to see a specialist who tells them there is nothing wrong and go away. They may go to another specialist who also tells them there is nothing wrong, go away, and the problem hasn't been dealt with. They still have the symptoms and they see you as the person who is unable to do anything for them even though they have been to hospital and had tests and it is easy in the hospital for you to say 'I realise you have pain in the eye but there is nothing structurally wrong with the eyeball, back to doctor.' Perhaps vice versa when we do things and achieve things, it is OK, you don't always hear something about it, whereas if you are in a certain sort of speciality, results are much more instant. It is associated with much more respect.

On bad days

I felt I was the dustbin of human society and thinking back it sounded a horrible thing to say but I must have felt it at that time to say that because anything that went wrong was your fault and anything that went wrong in hospital was your fault as well. You felt you were taking on sort of everybody else's worries and concerns and this is one of the things I do find with general practice, although there are lots of nice things ... you feel manipulated. You also feel trapped because there is no let-out of it kind of feeling. I think that sometimes gets you. And the funny thing is, on the other side of the coin, I do know that I have very high satisfaction levels from my patients because we have done a sort of qualitative research analysis using validated things and it is very high and people like me, but unfortunately, for some reason, this small element of sort of dissatisfaction seems to take away a lot of the goodness about it. I think it probably does because you feel you can't afford to be perfect all the time. And if I was in hospitals I could be because I could do a series of this and this and this and say 'nothing to do with your eyes, nothing to do with your gastro-enterology system', after somebody else because the structures are not laid down, whereas a lot of the things we see are very nebulous and they don't fit into any of these criteria and they perhaps actually don't have a beginning and an end either.

He recently met another student friend from medical college who couldn't believe he was a GP, working in 'a backwater'. It reminded him of how trivial some of the role could be: 'like writing out, the consultant this morning in the clinic at the hospital instead of giving a prescription out to the patient he will say, go around to the surgery and ask them to give you a prescription for this and I am tempted to take that personally ...' But a consultant paediatrician had sat with him in surgery and was surprised at the complexity of the work. 'He had felt lost with regard to what I was doing, whereas I was able to swing through what he was doing bar one or two technical sides like putting in a tube into a baby's trachea.'

The research finished more or less where we began, with his father:

Thinking back now, actually, considering what a strong character my father was and how not so strong I was, thinking back now, I think it was actually a big thing to do at that time although at that time I wasn't aware of breaching any thing, or I wasn't actually aware of the fact that I was making my own mark, but I think perhaps there might have been a little bit of that because ... initially obviously there was pressure for me not to proceed with it and yet I did, and yet I have a very strong partner and a very strong family set-up. Thinking back I think maybe I was sort of making a point that I am my own person.

Moreover, had this been five years ago, Ambi said, ' I don't think I would have been so open because I was five years younger and I was going to set the world alight and sort everybody out. And no I wasn't going to let Linden see the inner side of me and I mean that. I wouldn't have been able to do so because the sort of, what I call the dark pride in me would have stopped me from revealing that.' His was a family, and this was a profession, in which what was inside was kept hidden away.

Mixed Messages

Greenhalgh and Hurwitz (1998) have argued that, over a long period, there has been 'a relentless substitution', of 'softer' skills of empathy, interpretation and subjective awareness with more 'scientific', objective and measurable values in the training of doctors. And that this partly reflects the power and utility of 'scientific objectivity' as a bureaucratic benchmark for defining what works and why. Expertise becomes separated from expert, knowledge from knower, and doctors ought to make similar judgements in roughly the same set of circumstances. Contrariwise, of course, questions are being asked about whether medicine is a science at all, and there is the burgeoning alternative and complementary medicine movement where the softer and human skills are greatly valued. There are many views on the role of science in medicine and there may be a danger – in emphasising the neglect of the softer and human skills – of forgetting some of the benefits of scientific medicine, in, for example, the better care and management of chronic disease (Burton, 2000). The problem remains, however, of the normalising power of 'big science'.

Dr John Sadler defined himself as a 'feminine' doctor with a strong psychological, more specifically psychoanalytic, orientation. He had never felt omnipotent. He had a deep interest in the spiritual aspects of the work too, as well as in the wider socially aware medicine. John was distressed by present trends, by the power of evidence-based medicine, narrowly conceived, and the influence of what he termed 'the Royal College agenda'. If the future was uncertain he feared the struggle for a more psychologically literate profession was being lost. He felt, increasingly, out of tune with a world that valued quick, cheap solutions, certainties and crude measurement. Health managers wanted simple formulae and precise audits of the costs and benefits of heath care. Subtlety was no longer prized. General practice and primary care were driven by crude economic criteria.

In Flux

John was Balint-trained. He was committed to his professional and personal development and aspired to being more of an academic. He once hoped to become a trainer in general practice but had abandoned this ambition because he was unsure of himself as a teacher. He used a diverse range of therapies in his practice and was constantly trying out new ones, including acupuncture. He loved stories too and was the sort of person who had no worry in talking of personal matters:

> Whereas when I listen to men speaking, the locker-room talk, I think it is a load of males banging their chests around ... but I am actually quite comfortable about speaking with women about personal issues. I think I have got a lot of feminine aspects to my personality which I am not ashamed of and my anima is quite strong, I recognise that. I know I am hairy and big and strong and go to the gym ... but I am quite prepared to admit that my, the yin side of me, is developed. I am quite energetic. My yang side is quite developed, but there are a lot of feminine aspects of me, which I am quite happy about, traditionally feminine ... I don't mind opening up to people. My whole family is like that.

John believed that many of the inter-personal messages, which were so influential at one stage in general practice, were being sidelined as GPs became 'pseudo scientists, measurers and counters; psychological perspectives have actually gone by the wayside'. This was a disaster. Statistics, however well collected and whatever larger story they might tell, were never as complex as individuals:

> ... The profession is very masculine. I refuse to engage in that. I am not powerful. I appear to be powerful. I can project, I can hypnotise people, I can stick needles in people, I can project myself. I can act powerful, but I know it is the Wizard of Oz, all done by smoke and mirrors. I am happy with that. It is a sham. That plays to the sham within me. It is this, I like that, I like that.

The sham is that it is all a game of soldiers, it doesn't matter. Underneath we are people ... we are all souls and we are all together. There is no difference between you and me fundamentally we are imperfect beings in an imperfect world trying to get better.

The Royal College

Science was about power:

So we are talking about people having power over things that are difficult. Disease and illness is difficult to cope with, for society to cope with, so we give it to the most powerful people, the scientists. We don't want these namby-pamby therapists and what have you coping with diseases that can kill us and things like this. What do they know? Any decent journalist would make mincemeat of a therapist, but not of a scientist. It is this sort of thing I think. Society wants powerful people involved ... It is a load of crap ... It is a load of crap, it is a buzzword. Believe me, evidence-based. If you want evidence-based medicine you won't practise medicine. Because most of what we do is not evidence-based. I can give placebos. OK you want evidence-based medicine why the hell do we give drugs, why don't we give placebos to everybody as first time medicine because we know that 30 per cent of people will respond to a placebo for anything. Why don't people use placebos? That is evidence, let us use that. Evidence-based medicine is a way of cost containment I think. It is the Royal College ... they won, there was the Balint lot and the Royal College. I was a supporter of the College but I am very doubtful. We got sold down the river by the College. We have now become pseudo scientists ... Actually science is the buzzword; if you want funding, or if you want to be taken seriously you become a scientist. The College is seen as scientific and it got in with the Government, seen as a way of pushing the profession from the BMA, became polarised between the College and the BMA and we got the scientist so-called measure and it fits in with the Government way of measuring things. It has all become very political. Basically science means measuring and what we are doing in medicine is measuring, we are measuring care, we are using performance indicators and there is nothing wrong in that in its place. Evidence, evidence to what, if you show that medicine ... You might be able to show that there is evidence that doctors don't do anything at all. Let's get rid of the doctors. May even be that. I don't mind. I could do something else. I could write science fiction.

A patient came to mind, at that moment, and John smiled:

> Did I tell you about the story about the guy on his wedding night? I
> thought I had. I was in this practice and this Nigerian bloke came in
> and it was his wedding night and he was worried about impotence.
> Young, fit man, nothing to worry about at all. Had lots of anxieties and
> this man was very intelligent, worked hard, Ph.D. and he wanted me to
> give him something for his wedding night and I said 'Well hang on a
> minute.' If I was in Nigeria, and I don't know, but I assume that this
> would be standard, accepted practice and I have got the very thing for
> you. So in the cupboard we had some alkaline and some, a white
> mixture, when you mix them together they foam and they go into this
> milky fluid. I mixed it before his eyes, it foamed and I said 'It looks like
> semen.' He said 'Yes' and I said 'If you take that then you won't have
> any problems.' Gave it to him and the next week he came back, shook
> me by the hand and he went like this, 'Thank you so much doctor, it
> was very very effective ...'

The Scientist

Strange that he felt so strongly about science and its more grandiose
tendencies, he said, because he trained as a scientist:

> I have a science degree and my inclination is towards science, but I think
> I am scientific enough to know that the job I am doing isn't particularly
> scientific, and that attempting to dress it up as such is often ... everybody
> turns to science to justify what they do. That is what Freud did,
> considered himself to be a scientist, but he wasn't. I see that happening
> in medicine but I think sometimes you lose something in the measuring.
> I don't know. I will tell you how I see it. I look back to when apothe-
> caries and surgeons and physicians didn't consider themselves to be in
> the same profession. I see what is happening now when we have nurse
> practitioners who are not sure whether they are nurses or doctors and I
> look towards the twenty-first century and just wonder if what we see in
> the medical profession is really a transient phase, as it was before the
> apothecaries etc. came together as one profession. I wonder if we will
> all change. I am now working closely with osteopaths and practice
> nurses so I am one of these people who like to take a broader, cosmic
> view of things, but I don't know what one's role is any more. I used to
> know it was to see people and to look after them.
>   And the things I am interested in like the social problems and the
> counselling, I don't have the time for and that gives me a sinking feeling

inside, because I know I don't have time – I send them to a counsellor. So I am not quite sure what I am. I know the person I am, I know what motivates me, but am not quite sure what kind of doctor I am. Which is why I chose not to become a trainer, when I had been on the trainers' course, because I didn't want to inflict my uncertainty on people. Perhaps I am not a very good teacher as I have discovered. I get carried away. I don't know, I am confused, but I am not pessimistic, because there are certain things that happen ... it is very difficult when you are tired to take stock of your life ... I have developed back pain, which I have had for the last year, which I am sure has a large psychological element in it. I don't know. Right now I know I am having osteopathy and Alexander technique therapy. I am doing that at the moment, in an attempt to straighten myself out.

Frustration

He was happy with certain aspects of change: the convergence, for instance, of the nurse and GP's role. There was a possibility, he thought, that in due course, nurse practitioners and doctors might be taught from a common syllabus. Nurses were often better at the technical side, teaching people about asthma techniques, monitoring their asthma or diabetes, for instance. They were enthusiastic, he said, about the protocols, because it is new for them. He was bored with it. He was interested in the doctor/patient relationship, and responding to ill-health in diverse ways, and in partnership with his patients:

What I do find upsetting and amazing, is that they are still discussing in medical schools about the role of teaching the consultation to medical students. I have probably said this before. I went to a medical school where we had training with actors who were method actors and they explained how they felt about the thing. We got feedback and we did it again until we got it right. That is still considered to be avant-garde, but I went to medical school in the early Seventies and they are still being discussed. I am absolutely amazed. I understand that at Barts they are just introducing this, if they are introducing it at all. I find that just very odd ... where I was is no longer a new medical school and surely these things have been disseminated widely, but obviously they haven't.

Consolations

These were hard times John said, for a doctor like him. He was not happy, and sought consolation in writing. He would like to write a book but lacked confidence to do so, just now. He had a strong creative urge, a desire to make things work. This was his antidote to depression:

> I don't know, I don't know. Control, control; anxiety; insecurity. My father was ill with rheumatoid arthritis for a long time and that is why I became a doctor, I think. My sister is very insecure, she's four years younger than me and she is more insecure than I was. I got at least four years of the good days before Dad became ill, but it's a strong sense of insecurity. My mother is insecure – her mother was ill and her parents died when she was young, so this is, again it's a familial thing – insecure mother who then finds herself in a situation where her husband was ill, the children are insecure, and I ended up as a doctor. There's all sorts of things going on there. So that is where the obsessiveness comes from; wanting to be in control. I've always had this feeling of strength through adversity that you can turn anything to good use. I used to call it worry-power when I was a kid, I used to use my worry-power to get myself through my exams ...
>
> ... My dad is a lovely man, but he is not the strong father, he is not the strong parental figure. My dad is quite emotional, not weak, not a weak man, but vulnerable. My mum was always the one, the strong person in the family. So I am aware of taking other powerful male figures' agendas ... I was seven when he lost his job. I think I must have been about four when he became ill. That is a very formative time. My sister of course, she never saw the good times and so she is very much more insecure than me. And again it is all to do with what happens at home. What happened at home. It is interesting because I don't like illness. I really don't. My mum is not comfortable with illness and yet here I am surrounded by sick people. Everyone I know. My sister has got ulceric colitis. My neighbour who is an interesting chap, a very high-powered man, he is now disabled and he lives in his swimming pool. Everybody I know, in some way, my friend's girl friend who he has just split up with, she had ME. I mean everybody I know is ill. Not just my patients. And I feel sometimes like it is closing in on me. So when I get ill I get very, very upset ... I had a cold, I had tinnitus, right, Dad has got tinnitus. So why I am a doctor? The man is frightened of illness and yet he is dealing with sick people all the time. It is doing what you don't like. Learning to love the enemy. Overcoming your fears I think.

We exchanged stories of being men and of feeling vulnerable, in his case, in medicine, and, in mine, in academe. We talked about our research relationship and of his need to prove himself to me, transferentially. Knowing something of psychodynamics, I was able to offer insights into the paternal roots of the transference. But there were no easy solutions to our shared and wider struggle to build more emotional literacy in what still remains, in large part, a 'real man's' world.

9
Cultures of Silence

> The important lesson is to learn to watch for what is not being said, and to consider the meanings of silences.
>
> Paul Thompson, *The Voice of the Past*

Minority Sport?

It has been suggested, time and again, that psychological knowledge and emotional literacy have never been given sufficient priority in the medical world. Yet doctors are living, experiencing people, and patients impact on their inner lives. Recent research (Cape, 1996) suggests there is little application by doctors of psychotherapeutic ideas, even of brief psychotherapy, to the patient/doctor interaction or to their own feelings and professional development. Andrew Elder (1999) considers interest in psychological medicine among GPs to be 'a minority sport'. Participation in Balint-type groups, specifically designed to enable GPs to manage the emotional dimensions of their work, is minority sport too. Many GPs believe an understanding of patients' emotional conflicts and their connections to physical illness, as well as their impact on patient and doctor interactions, are marginal to the real business of medics. They belong to the counsellor rather than themselves (Balint et al., 1993).

The problem is, in part, cultural; the difficulty of talking to colleagues about disturbed or troubled feelings when things go wrong and a doctor feels uncertain and inadequate. It can be considered, for good empirical reasons, detrimental to a career to admit mental distress. The present chapter illustrates that, even when GPs engage in Balint groups and consider, in depth, the emotional dynamics of the work, issues surrounding the interplay of personal and professional identities tend to be omitted from the conversation, even when crucial to the performance of the role. This is partly for fear of what others might think and say.

144

Hard Work

Dr Rose Clarke had moved to her new practice, after an unhappy, occasionally traumatic time in her previous partnership. The problems she experienced were not simply to do with patients and their material poverty. Her partners in the practice did not talk to each other. Attempts were made at group learning, but this was resisted. Some partners thought there was real work to be done, rather than sitting around with their feet up for half an hour, drinking coffee:

> It was felt that, they tried it before and there wasn't enough time to do that. So it was suggested that we meet up once a month in the evening and have a meal and talk to each other and then one of the partners said he didn't think his wife would like us meeting up for a meal, so it was cut down to 'Well, we will meet up one evening a month', and that for me is just not enough communication ... And I felt the way that the practice dynamics worked there, there was a good practice manager, but a very powerful practice manager who I think, well I know, had a lot of problems of her own, and very child-like behaviour. And as with most children she didn't like people saying no and if they said no she had the equivalent of an adult tantrum. Consequently I realised that the partners had always just done what she wanted them to do for five years and it meant that it was very difficult to do anything. You would suggest something and well OK if you speak to so and so about it, which would be the practice manager and you would have to liaise with her and nothing happened.

Colleagues were hiding from each other, and from the manager, in a culture of silence.

Peculiar Practice

Rose talked of medicine as a world in which confidentiality and boundaries were permeable:

> Yes basically when I did psychiatry I worked for a consultant who was labelled by everybody as a psychopath. He had various complaints against him and after I finished the job that job was removed from the GP training scheme. And while I was doing the job I became very, very unhappy. I became depressed and instead of saying that I actually took two weeks off with flu. But it was, it was dreadful, particularly doing psychiatry and feeling so awful yourself. And at the time I felt it was

directly related to doing the job. In retrospect I think that was the final straw.

... he was a very, very difficult man to work for. And also I didn't like the way he was with the patients. I didn't feel, I have to be very careful because I don't want to slander someone else.

... Yes, but I didn't feel that he valued the patients. I didn't feel that he respected the patients. I mean his first question to any patient whether they were schizophrenic, depressed or – what is your sex life like? And this as an opening line ... in a grand ward round.

No one had warned or spoken to her about his ways. There was the power, too, of the consultant's patronage: a career could be irreparably damaged if the wrong things were said. It was dangerous to talk in this hierarchical world.

Personal Depression

Rose became clinically depressed and sought help. Unfortunately, her colleagues in the practice found out about her problems and confidentiality was breached:

I don't know. I will never know how it got back, but basically, having sought help, which is a very difficult thing to do, that lifeline was then cut off. And so my GP actually arranged something totally unconventional which was actually perfect and that is why I will do things differently for other people. You take a certain amount of risk. She took a risk. If you don't record everything in the notes. If you don't do things by the book, medically and legally you take a risk, but I will take that risk ... My personal belief is that I think a lot of doctors have been or are depressed, are or have been suicidal and they can't face up to it. That is my explanation for it. That most people when they go through, either as a medical student, or when they qualify or then when they get their general practice, or they get themselves a job, run into problems. And they find it very difficult to get help and talk to people about it ... I think first of all, particularly for doctors, access to health care is actually very difficult. It is very difficult. It is OK if you are going about your big toe nail, but it is very difficult to get a confidential service. Because we talk about confidentiality, computers, telephone calls, letters, and I think doctors, of all people, are aware of despite how careful we are with confidentiality that sometimes slip-ups occur. And doctors are aware of the life insurance and all those sort of things, so they won't go and get help for things. Well if I have something wrong with me, which fortunately at the moment I am not aware that I have, then I wouldn't want to go and consult a doctor. So I had ... I wasn't going to go and consult a doctor because that will be on my form and that is going to load my life insurance. So I think we have more awareness and I think also as a profession our colleagues do actually kill themselves and I think we find it very difficult to deal with that. There has been a suicide ... last year, and that has never really been dealt with. People don't really mention it.

... they don't want to dwell on it. And there is also a lot of guilt because our colleagues do kill themselves, they do become alcoholics, they do have drug problems. I think also there is, I know particularly, I know with this particular person everyone would say, 'Well I saw him and I didn't realise', so there is all the guilt with that that there was someone working amongst them who no one realised was struggling so much.

Rose had a good GP friend who committed suicide. Colleagues had not been as helpful or accessible as they might have been. People will, at a superficial level, express concern but actually want, in the pressured environment of the surgery, the partner back at work. It was their individual responsibility, in effect, to cope. Everyone struggled, at times, and suffered; it was part of the job, something to be managed and/or suffered in silence, a private more than a professional concern. GPs, in the inner-city, are under so much stress, Rose insisted, that if a practice is one person down, 'that can sometimes be enough just to make the whole partnership fold up. And it does happen in some partnerships. You have one off sick and another one goes off sick, and it all gets too much to cope with.'

Balint

Balint groups have represented one significant way for many GPs to manage the emotional demands of their work, even if only ever a minority (Balint et al., 1993). Paul Sackin (1994) has described the key principles underlying the work. There is normally a leader with some psychoanalytic, group analytic or equivalent training, working with eight or nine doctors. The material for the group derives from current cases (as in the work of the SDL groups described earlier). The focus for discussion is the relationship between the doctor and her patient; and there is a great stress on confidentiality and openness as well as respect for all group members. The basic purpose of the group is to increase understanding of patients' problems, not to find solutions. The intention is to create a reflexive, collaborative space for learning.

Balint groups wrestle with the basic paradox of being a GP in which the most characteristic aspects of the role are hard to define. It is made up of bits of everything (gynaecology, cardiology and so on) but also the 'accessible generalist' must resist easy definitions. Too early a focus may inhibit the development of a deeper perspective connecting the different parts of the patient's narrative and symptomatology together. Time is also needed to understand how the doctor and patient relate one to another, and, through this, to establish how useful different kinds of medical intervention may be (Balint et al., 1993). General practice is, at core, about the management of uncertainty and learning how to both live with and learn from it.

Balint groups were never intended for personal therapy although self-awareness may increase as a result of involvement (Sackin, 1994). Discomfort or distress in the doctor are not ignored but are worked through in the context of considering the needs and problems of the patient. Michael Balint himself was clear that doctors could usefully be in therapy themselves and that the prime focus of the group was the patient and the relationship with the doctor, rather than the psychological difficulties of the doctor which should be dealt with elsewhere (Balint, 1957). But the boundary is problematic and aspects of the doctor's own history and identity can be crucial to understanding the doctor/patient dynamic and yet may be omitted from the story for other reasons. Balint groups in mainland Europe appear to be more flexible in considering the interplay of the personal and the professional in telling stories about the consultation.

In the Minority

Colin Smith is of the earnest minority active in Balint groups. Colin Smith is also gay and had never talked of his sexuality in a Balint group, despite its importance in the consulting room and in relationships with particular patients. Our conversations raised uncomfortable and 'muddled feelings' for him; about a tendency to feel overly detached from some patients and perhaps from his personal history and private self too. There was unfinished business, he said, to do with his family and its difficult emotional dynamics.

The importance of Balint to his learning and professional development was clear from the outset. His self-perception as a doctor came from working and learning in Balint groups. He had been active in them from when first a trainee and found it hard to imagine how someone could have a firm idea of the basis of professional behaviour without such involvement:

Well the GP that I was a trainee with had been in a Balint group, but also the vocational training course I was on included a weekly Balint group in the second half of the afternoon ... One of the reasons I went to train with him, very odd experience, I came to London one day to find a training practice and for some reason went into his house, and we instantly got on to psychosomatic medicine and it wasn't anything that he had ever studied in medical school. Because in England you don't study psychosomatic medicine basically in medical school but it must have come out of my mouth and it was like, you know, here's the place because there was a meeting of minds about that and he was very interested in that sort of thing. That leads into Balint because the work of Balint groups deals with the frustration that GPs originally had after the war with non-medical problems that they were presented with. And of course medical problems that they couldn't do anything about because there was so much less that you could do about it I think. And so maybe my practice has always been skewed a bit that way.

A First Group

He talked about being in a group:

> ... I wasn't desperate to go to it, but it was something that grew a bit on you, talking in detail about people. It was an area where it was valid to talk about how you felt about people, about patients and about the idea that general practice could include that sort of thing because it is not something you ever talk about at medical school and I suppose a little bit like psychotherapy ... the first time that you are allowed this space to talk about things. And it lets those things assume the importance they probably really have ... it gives you space to talk about the side of your career, what your job is about, both about the patients and about the things about being a doctor, about what doctors do and what doctors don't do.

Colin said that, even now, he often felt nervous when talking about Balint:

> Very nervous of being glib about things and obviously the impression I make and as always with people who have been involved in Balint work in England. I feel embarrassed about it as if it is something, something naughty you do, a bit like English people would talk about their psychotherapy experiences.

Colin was also aware that Balint, as well as the research, raised questions for him about therapy. He was reticent about talking too openly with GP colleagues:

> I was conscious again today and also on reading the things that maybe I talk, I talk more than I think I would in this kind of situation and I talk maybe only about the things I want to talk about, but I am not sure about that. I am very conscious that I have an on-going thing about therapy and the fact that I imagine I wouldn't be able to talk for an hour, but I can quite easily see that I would have no problems whatsoever and might be completely addicted to it, which is strange. But obviously the other people, part of the reason why you have been able to interview doctors like this is because we don't mind doing that, or some of us want to do that I guess. Want to be able to reflect.
>
> ... You can view a Balint group as a qualitative research tool because it is a group of people who meet together and talk about issues and generate material that could be analysed, which is actually the way Balint groups work. The books about general practice, about doctor–patient relationship are derived in that way by someone studying transcripts of Balint groups and amassing the information and trying to work out what it means. And in the last three years we have had a Balint group that is meeting to try and look at 'doctors' defences'. About the way you defend yourself against patients or how you get into funny situations with patients because of past experience and it does end up, we are ending up talking a bit about the doctors' personal experiences themselves as well as just their professional stance, which is something that Balint groups in England have tried not to deal with because traditionally it was thought to be rather difficult and might end up making the groups into personal therapy groups.

Counter-transference

Balint groups had generated insights into his 'counter-transference' and its significance in certain encounters. Counter-transference involves the doctor's, perhaps unconscious, responses to a patient. The counter-transference represents, in therapy, vital clinical evidence, and a crucial means to understanding the patient's inner-world, how s/he might be feeling and the doctor–patient interaction (Samuels, 1993). Colin talked of certain patients:

> A patient of mine that we talked about a lot was someone who appeared a very self-confident, youngish man, forties, appeared fit and healthy,

but when I saw him he both had sort of asthma and described his life as being totally lacking in any pleasure or joy and there is something about that in me ... There was certainly an element of my consultations which avoided talking about that sort of thing but I have some sort of fear of, well fear of life being, something being taken away in life, or of it not being happy, and of appearing to be one thing, but actually being another. Another issue that sometimes comes up with patients of mine is I sometimes get a lot of trouble with certain kinds of female patients, people like my step-mother ... and I have a weird business about over-compensating or feeling like not compensating and getting rather angry and sometimes over-compensating and being terribly nice to them in an inappropriate way ... There is a whole element that are professional defences ... but then there is also a layer of personal things ... and it is not an area that has been written a lot about ... This could be me, and you tend to over-protect patients like that. You do things that you, beyond the call of duty perhaps, that aren't particularly useful ... For instance this particular guy was apparently a successful businessman ... I gave him actual tablets from my drawer. Anti-depressants, rather than writing a prescription I actually gave him tablets and it was an odd thing for me to do, but I had some and I gave them to him. I was unhappy to give him tablets, but I try and gloss over the unhappiness, or hope it would go away...there is some resonance between the two of you that stops you really being objective.

... Beware of a doctor. You are talking to a doctor and then they suddenly start examining you or taking your blood pressure because it probably means they are ... thinking hard which I felt with this guy that I was thinking hard. I started listening to his chest because I was trying to digest what he was saying, but it is also true that I was probably trying to cut off what he was saying, by doing something very medical, because then you feel like you are being a proper doctor.

Distinguishing what most appropriately belongs to the patient and what to the therapist is a core issue in psychotherapy, and, it seems, in general practice, as is understanding why particular patients have such a strong and occasionally disturbing impact. Balint enabled Colin to understand the potential power of such dynamics in his professional life and how conventional distinctions between self and other were, on occasions, blurred. The biggest challenge, he said, was to sort out what belonged to the patient and what to the doctor; and this raised large questions about the place of the personal and autobiographical in Balint-type groups.

The Personal and the Professional

Colin wondered, over the course of the research, about introducing more personal material in Balint groups:

> ... You shouldn't say too much that is personal. Whereas talking about defences has certainly brought up personal things because the way you behave to people has to do with your self and your professional self and so it has been forced to come out. We are aware that in other countries where Balint groups are more successful, such as in Germany and France, perhaps the personal things are talked about more in the groups and we are wondering whether that may be a way; and that maybe in 2000 British doctors might be, Balint groups might work better in Britain if there was a bit more personal revelation, personal talking in them. That this objective 'I'm a doctor, this is my patient' suited the mid-fifties in England perhaps very well when doctors were, or people in general were, quite loath to express their personal feelings, but maybe nowadays people might be attracted to a slightly more, a group where you were, where there was more freedom to talk about personal problems.
>
> ... People would be, you know if someone started to say, 'Well you know my mother was beaten by my father', the group leader would say, 'Well that is not really our area', we should talk about the case, which I think has a validity because it does, it takes it away a bit. It makes the group more orientated towards the doctor and helping the doctor rather than helping the patient perhaps, because you are looking at more what is the problem for the doctor rather than the patient. You are looking at the doctor end of the doctor–patient relationship, more than the patient end, whereas traditionally you try to stay in the middle, or towards the patient end.

Family History

Colin talked of his family that had been 'high on anxiety'. His parents did not get on at all well and Colin, wanted, always, to put things right:

> It was serious. They split up when I was eighteen in the end and I suppose, it is interesting because we didn't know about it as there was a lot of dishonesty going on as well. My father was being actually dishonest in terms of lying about what he was doing, that sort of thing ...
>
> ... I think he may have done things outside the house that were not relationships. I don't know quite what he did, but my mother still lies

to herself emotionally about what things, what was the situation and what she wanted, or was willing to do about it.

Moreover, he said, being gay did not mean that he was a 'touchy feely', emotionally empathic doctor:

Maybe gay people are in general quite happy to keep their distance I think.

... I think it is more like to do with, yes to do with medical culture in that medical culture makes you scared of patients knowing too much about you and that sort of thing, perhaps.

... I find it, yes, I find it amazing to think that young male doctors have to deal with attractive female patients really frequently and how they deal with that considering the turmoil it causes me if I have to deal with a young, attractive male patient which is a much rarer thing. I don't mean turmoil, I mean that it brings issues up, the fact that you have got, that male doctors are examining, doing intimate examinations, which of course is much more common to do intimate examinations on female patients. It must be, there must be amazing things going on inside.

... I suppose that sort of abuse, sexual abuse by doctors, is the tip of it. The tip of that undealt-with business. Yes, it is a big subject and I do think about it because I think being able to talk about it is important. I think it must be better to say you saw someone recently you were very sexually attracted to, rather than just feel it. I think it must be ... But I am not sure. Maybe it just makes you more aware of things if you say them, but I think it tends to – I think for me it certainly works the other way round. Express something like that, it desexualises it doesn't it?

Colin defined himself as a practical doctor. He often felt impatient with the woolliness and subjectivity of social science:

I have done a social science module ... the sociology of medicine, is really a descriptive thing ... It is not a problem-solving discipline thing I don't think ... the lecturer, the guy who was teaching was purported to be very hands off, you know, not that social scientists should be in charge of lots of social policy but that they can investigate and provide information for social policy makers, which seemed important to me because of reading so much social science material. It is so heavily laden with people's political or their own judgements. It is not at all, well you very rarely seem to get writers who are very unbiased. Most people seem to be very biased so if they are making decisions that are completely along their political lines or the lines that they think. It is interesting because the Balint work is also, compared to almost anything else in general practice, is un-problem-oriented. You are not there in the group to solve problems. Ostensibly you may do so by elucidating things in other ways. Yes, like psychodynamic therapy it is not there necessarily solving the problem.

He had been taught to be objective and yet general practice was muddled and unclear; partly therapy, partly medicine, partly sociology. He was probably avoiding psychological issues in his life history too:

It is funny, I was just thinking today my friend who is someone I went out with when we were in medical school, has been in analysis, she was in analysis for about eight years and she is now this year starting a, she took twenty years to qualify as a doctor but is now going to become a psychiatrist and is starting her training analysis and it is something ... Balint has become a passion in that same sort of way, fulfilling some need but maybe like we have been talking about is a bit removed, that I have never wanted to go into analysis or have personal psychother-apy but I am very happy to be in a situation where I think about that sort of thing a lot, about one's own perceptions of people's feelings. And try and analyse yours and theirs and think about them is a situation I like, but at a remove.

Yes, which is very interesting to think about because I imagine, I guess if I hadn't put myself in a forum, a place where I could talk about the way I felt about patients all the time, well over the years, probably I would have been in personal therapy. Because I don't know what I would have done with all this material that comes at you over the years ...

... I can remember when I was a teenager, or early teens, twelve to fourteen, wanting to be a doctor to help people like my mother ... Because of her emotional difficulties but also she was a 'sickly person'.

He was making connections, with me, which he had not made before:

It feels like a beginning of something much longer. Because one has only been able to, as soon as you start to try and talk about things you realise how little you can really scratch the surface of what you really feel ... If you start to scratch the surface of personal problems, personal things for the doctor, if you started to do that you would just have a group of nine people. Patients would be just left behind probably because there is so much there that even if you are feeling relatively secure and successful as I think I am at the moment, compared to other times in my life, I still, as soon as you start talking about it you think of things. But you don't tie this sort of thing up very well and even if you had some sort of psychotherapy for five years or something you still wouldn't probably achieve some tying-up of anything to do with opening up and perhaps, from day to day, I suppose in life in many things I am very much someone who wants to tie things up and have things and that is maybe why I don't want to open up a lot of psychological issues and I certainly practise it in day-to-day life. You can see how tidy all this is, maybe that is crazy because that is not the way my work really is, because actually there are all sorts of things going on all the time, continuing, but I like it to appear like, I like to shut each patient down in my mind. I dictate every letter right after the surgery so I don't go on thinking about them.

... I just think that there are several patients that I would just like to cut the crap and talk a bit more with them about other things ...

... And in this kind of practice in this part of London it doesn't happen that often. But I can imagine if you worked in Hampstead it must be a whole different thing where there would be lots of patients and you would like to be their friends ... I think I have mentioned this before in these interviews about GPs that select themselves to work in places like this, must be people that want to be defended against relationships with their patients in some way, because it is often the GPs who are training to work in this area who will say – I couldn't stand the idea of meeting Mrs Bloggs in the High Street or the idea of treating another doctor as a patient and this kind of thing horrifies them ... it is a funny thing because it is taking on the world but not in a personal way. Yes it is exactly that, take on all these immigrants and all this kind of thing but it is not, it is taking on a, it is at a remove again. It is taking on the world at quite a remove like the, what you call it, going to Africa ... preaching religion. Yes a missionary it is a position of great power but a long way away from the people you are seeing.

Good Practice

Relationships between colleagues can be a source of salvation. Patricia Johnstone had known good and bad practices. She now worked in a group practice committed to cultural and psychological literacy and among colleagues who helped her negotiate a major crisis.

'Disturbance disturbs,' she said. There was a woman patient, with four children, whose husband was murdered in front of her and the children in Kurdistan. The patient was looking after the children, on her own, in a tower block. She was isolated and the trauma of what had happened was only just beginning to manifest itself. She came to the doctor complaining: 'I have too much headache, I get headache when the children cry and I shout at them.' Social Services tried to help by providing a secondhand cooker:

... which was so filthy and leaked gas that she had to pay somebody a fiver to get rid of it. Now I can say to her that I don't want to hear any of that because that is not medical, that is social services, but actually all that is tied up in this whole stress thing. She is presenting with headaches, the headaches are very much stress-related. How do you disentangle all of that? You might write yet another letter to Social Services, but how do you actually change things? I feel incredibly cynical about this society that people can do that to people with that degree of poverty that they can be given a leaking, totally filthy cooker as being our society's response to somebody in dire straits having no way of cooking food for her children.

The boys were behaving badly and the youngest was 'acting out' at school. He wanted to tell his friends about what had happened to his dad. But he would burst into tears and could not speak. The children needed to talk but the mother was stopping them. This distressed Patricia. And she had also to deal with a serious complaint from a patient:

I ended up doing examinations for cancer on anything that moved, for a while! If there was the slightest reason for doing it. I calmed down from all of that and actually got back to where I think I had been before, which was practising fairly safe medicine and actually as time went by I changed a lot immediately after it, but I think actually what I had been doing was fairly safe before that anyway and there were issues around the woman, for instance not coming back for a follow-up, and then there was never anything to actually tell you that this was something more serious.

She was sued and being able to talk to her partners was critical to survival. Pat had felt lost in the role for a while:

I was easily stressed by it. I was often very stressed by work. I suppose I felt a mixture of things. I felt resentful that it was taking up so much time. I had wanted for a while before that to reduce my hours, but it took a while before we could arrange it here. I didn't blame anybody that it took that length of time, because it actually does take some time to set up alternatives. I suppose I felt a bit frustrated occasionally that it was taking that length of time. I was aware of the fact when I had come back from holiday, so when I had had a break, I was aware of how much more I enjoyed the job and I felt was more useful to patients. And I could see the contrast between that and the extreme which would be when I was coming up to needing a holiday, but not even that extreme, but just not being newly back from holiday and feeling fresh. I could feel that I was often just stale and would be short with patients and then feel bad about that, about being short with patients. I think that was it really. I wasn't interested in doing any kind of reading. I had had it up to here, I don't want anything else. That was my feeling.

The death of a close friend finally brought matters to a head:

I used to feel very much like I was stepping into a role and used to feel like a role before that and I felt I was me interacting with you the patient, and yes, OK, I was a doctor and had a whole load of things, but also I was me as a person. And I think it was integrating those two bits. I stopped thinking compartmentalised. I had always been compartmentalised, whether it was this thing about growing up, a foreigner in Britain, don't let them know what you are thinking. There is all this sort of separation bit. I used to, my friends used to laugh at the clothes I wore when I was working in hospitals – shoes; I wore these, as they call them, 'lady doctor' shoes. I would push on some kind of a uniform almost, it wasn't a particular uniform but it was very unlike clothes that I wore any other time and I justified wearing them, well they were covered up with a white coat and actually it was something to do with the uniform, so that people wouldn't realise that I shouldn't be there. That kind of thing ... I think it was being Welsh and a woman. Yes, it was more as a woman, my counselling was really about the whole negative thing about woman – femaleness – and not being worthy, that sort of whole thing. So yes the Welsh bit as well. The people I found the most terrifying in my twenties were English women, the combination of the Welsh/English, and female. For a long time I always needed to make sure there were men around. I couldn't, I wouldn't choose to do anything with only women. Because although I wouldn't admit it I was actually petrified of them. So my counselling was very overdue and actually exceedingly effective. And I did not think of it in relation to work, but I noticed this huge change and it has made me far more confident, whether it is dealing with patients, dealing with partners, hospital, having to be the executive partner here. You know we take turns to be the executive partner. I am told by people that I am very good at covering it up. People don't realise that I am actually quaking and feeling completely unconfident. But it was just horrific the thought that I was going to have to do it. I remember doing it and people seemed to be quite happy with what I was doing, but feeling terrible. Now I have absolutely no problems. Once I had been through that process. I hadn't really tied the two up but when you see what else changed – that had changed before it, before the drop in time and I think my stress levels actually went down then, first of all. But the time involvement carried on with being very stressed. And then they went down again.

Working as she now did with caring colleagues made her feel 'like I am a different person. I know I am the same person but it felt such a huge change that it almost feels like I am a different person.'

This partnership contained people who had been going to therapists, were in therapy, and talked about it. So it was a culture anyway, where it was OK. And I don't remember that as being a problem at all and actually did talk to one of my partners about it, but in the time building up to it I think a few times I ended up talking to people, not because I wanted to, consciously, I wanted the ground to open up and swallow me, but because I had burst into tears. I felt in a totally unpredictable and completely overwhelming fashion. They were always very good the way they dealt with it and I found it excruciatingly embarrassing. So that was already happening and I felt it was happening despite myself, and I still didn't do anything about it. It almost didn't really happen, wasn't really me, was the way I handled it.

Pat was continually anxious about sharing her story and carefully edited the transcripts. She did not want to reveal too much to particular colleagues in the area who would only criticise or ridicule what was said. Her immediate colleagues were the exception, to prove a rule in a culture in which silence was most often the wisest option.

10
Performing and Underperforming

On a huge hill, cragged and steep, truth stands, and hee that will reach her, about
must, and about must goe;
And what the hill's suddenness resists, winne so;

John Donne, 'Satyre 111'

When I became General Manager of a Family Practitioners' Committee (as it then
was) in 1989, one of my first calls was from a woman GP who asked to see me
urgently. She arrived and started to tell me in detail about the (as she saw it) appalling
behaviour of her male professional partner. I was immediately struck by the similarity
of the language with that of ordinary relationship breakdowns, even to the point of
her saying at one point 'I thought he was going to hit me that morning' ... I waited
for the punch line, which I assumed was going to be that the partnership would be
breaking up, and began to wonder (as a new boy) what I would have to do. However
she just thanked me profusely for listening and prepared to leave. The only missing
line, I felt, was 'We're staying together for the sake of the patients.'

Malcolm Clarke

A Very Peculiar Practice

The health of some inner-city practices is frequently considered to be poor.
The pressure towards greater degrees of intervention in clinical
governance, and for a more extensive audit of GPs' performance seems,
in such contexts, irresistible. Some practices and services are shabby and
second-rate, by common consent. The issue is why and what to do about
it. The two case studies in this chapter illustrate what can go wrong but
also raise basic questions about the independent contractor status, as well
as the position and treatment of doctors from minority backgrounds.

Nothing had quite prepared Dr Rose Barker and a female colleague for
their new challenge in taking over an inner-city practice. There had been
no GP for over two years since the then single-hander retired:

It is outrageous Linden. A patient comes in, predominantly elderly
population ... people actually have very low expectations. They don't

want to disturb the doctor ... they are all on drugs that haven't been used for sort of fifteen years. And of course they are very traditional and they loved the old GP, but they are absolutely delighted that they have two new doctors, particularly two women doctors and I am very aware that to begin with I will be seen like the saviour on a white charger, but actually when push comes to shove and we try and institute change it may be difficult. It will be a difficult, slow process. So this group of patients, all of whom are actually very sick, you know. You go and visit people at home, there is diabetes uncontrolled that hasn't been looked at for two years. Most of the people that I visit have to go into hospital.

If the situation was grim, Rose and Kathy, her partner, were trying to respond positively to the 'challenge'. Rose was concerned at the chaos of the patients' notes, the pressure to sort out a lease, difficult patients to be seen and practical problems of telephones not working and computers crashing. The practice, moreover, had a locum from the old regime who was antagonistic towards the new partners. He had not been particularly well treated either by the Health Authority. But, whatever the justification, his attitude was a further burden to bear.

Exhilarated

Rose said she felt exhilarated as well as overwhelmed. She was 'excited with butterflies of excitement and delight on some days'. It was the first time either she or Kathy had run a practice. This was a new kind of learning: to run an organisation, manage people, design coherent systems of data storage and retrieval, and establish a warm and humane environment:

and I suppose it is learning to sort of remember that that is important ... And there are so many offshoots from that. Like we will be doing some teaching and hopefully it will be a university-linked practice, which means we will teach medical students and nurses. And we do plan to have some form of evaluation because everybody is very keen to sort of pilot what we are doing, so hopefully we will have somebody, an independent assessor who will come in and give us an ongoing appraisal and look at our education and personal needs. So that is being addressed as well because it can be very isolating you know.

There were mountains to climb in a socially deprived area:

Yes, white working class. Quite racist as well in some respects. Immigrant populations have come to the area and certainly my knowledge of the area was, because there was actually a very big, had a very big Greek community and my grandmother in fact historically got married in the area, met her husband in the area, so there are links, ironically. Yes. And I had actually worked in that area, again purely by chance, through my child health work, so I had covered that slot, that had been my slot ... you have had a number of immigrant populations that have come with the years. Most recently I suppose would be the Turkish population and now certainly some Africans, Ethiopians, Somalis, and some from Eastern Europe now. And there would appear to be a growing problem of homelessness. But you know there are no, there are very few residential houses. It is all estates. It is all high rise. It is all quite squalid actually, although behind the front door you then walk into actually lovely little houses, very nice little flats. Very nicely tended with little gardens and little flower pots. Very well cared for. So it is going to be an interesting mixture, very interesting mixed population.

There were low expectations of a doctor:

They all have these apocryphal stories about how Doctor Singh used to pop in and see them every week. I don't know how the man did it. I am sure he didn't. So that sort of feeling and everybody talks about Dr Singh who was one of the GPs that had the list who, you hear all the rumours that come out, that he used to be at work at ten o'clock at night with a bottle of whisky, so one patient said to me, which was an interesting insight. But he was the great hero and constantly being told that he was a lovely doctor, full stop. So the feeling that no matter what you do it will never be enough, no matter what you do you will always make mistakes. You will always be seen as the bad person. Yes, other problems are patients complaining about appointments and often they are very unfounded. If you are an emergency we will see you. It is just a feeling that you never do anything right Linden, just constantly battling and nobody really says thank you, well they do they do say thank you, but not often.
   ... I suppose the truth is you know that the Health Centre at the moment is such a poxy scum hole. I cannot describe it. I had to remove something today, looking for a pair of tweezers today. It took me twenty minutes to find a pair of tweezers. No equipment. There is nothing. Once I have my room set up and you know I have my plants and I have my pictures and pots and it is my room and you know we will have our computer and I will have some CDs and I will even have a bowl of fruit and some nice things that make it more homelike ...

Rose was taking lots of work home:

> ... I mean where do you start? Imagine that you have cabinets full of
> notes and any one, could be full of people who are just languishing at
> home with horrible illnesses. You just don't know because they are of
> the culture that they don't want to disturb the doctor. I went to see this
> bloke recently, seventy-five, I am not joking Linden, he was blue. He was
> blue and he has got this bad chest. He should have oxygen. He doesn't
> want it. So what can you do? He is making an informed choice about his
> life, but I have never seen a man so blue and able to walk around. So it
> is constant alarm really and I was sort of speaking to Kathy about it
> because Kathy isn't there at the moment. She doesn't start until February
> and I have to say it got to me a bit yesterday about, well what are we
> going to do here? How in heaven's name are we going to organise this?
> It is not that black. We have actually got, we are in the process of trying
> to recruit, a team of people who will come in and put the notes in order
> and put it all onto computer and ultimately in the next two years
> probably when we go and do visits we will just plug in a laptop into the
> phone line and access our computer. So we have got great dreams.

Rose and Kathy were putting together an administrative team consisting
of a practice manager, a practice nurse, a counsellor and others. She
wanted a multi-disciplinary group working effectively together in a
learning practice; a place in which time was set aside, every week, to
discuss, plan and learn in an open and egalitarian climate. Health care was
often a battle between warring tribes. The phones were not working either,
again, the day of the third interview and the new computing system had
crashed once more.

Six Months On

The practice moved from the 'poxy old slum' to a new health centre.
Managing staff had been a major preoccupation:

> There have been a couple of issues about some of the staff, that are a bit
> difficult and we are, I think they have a lot on their plate at the moment
> ... but we are worried that one is actually very much on a sort of work
> to rule, not that we want to work the guy into the ground but a little bit
> of greater flexibility would be nice.

Health Service bureaucracy had not helped either. The Health Authority,
in making the transfer of patients' names, wrongly allocated the majority
to her. Out of a list of 4,000, 3,500 went to Rose and she was swamped:

An error. An error. So any letter that came into the practice to do with any patient whether I knew them or not was stuffed in my pigeonhole because on the computer the name of the patient was allocated to me. I was the named doctor. So another cock up. What else? I mean there have always, there have always been unfortunately administrative errors made by other people and that is where you know, Kathy and I work fantastically as a team, we really do and maybe we are a bit obsessive about things but ...

Getting insurance for the new premises had been difficult. The alarm system, vital for security, had not worked and took five weeks to be repaired. Rose felt isolated, without proper support. The staff in the Health Authority, and in the various primary care teams, were too hard-pressed to help.

A Razor's Edge

She felt insecure, at times, about being a doctor:

You weren't prepared, you were taught all the causes ... you were taught the text books, but you weren't taught how to deal with very much else. How to be, what to be, how to deal with difficult patients. How to deal with anger, how to deal with dying. How to deal with all those emotional packages that come with the job. I don't think I was actually really prepared for that at all.

Particular patients pushed her to the edge:

You know people came in with a headache and you could almost bet your bottom dollar that they probably had a bloody intercranial tumour, or TB ... People are so sick, so ill ... People who had been tortured ... I had this one lady, Katie, and she was probably about my age and so there was, I don't know there was something in her that I think I probably empathised with. I definitely empathised. She had this older mother. She was completely neurotic, completely anxious. Julie came in with phenomenal somatisation problems, terribly anxious, never ever accepted any reassurance. Went to see one consultant after another and over the year I sort of developed a confidence with her, a good relationship with her, I think I was probably therapeutic in the sense that I was there as a familiar face that knew her and we would have a chat often. And I often used to think, surely there must be some psychotherapeutic technique that would help me ... Katie's mother had been ill and my mother was ill, is ill. Issues dealing with her anxieties about her mother. It is to do with empathy and boundaries and she did actually make me feel very uncomfortable at times and you know just an awareness of, I suppose, her anxieties. I felt that we were quite similar.

We spent time considering the patient within and why the previous practice had been allowed to deteriorate in such a way. Rose wondered about the importance of independent contractor status. She had to employ and manage staff, repair the building and security system as well as sort out the chaos of patients with the wrong notes and outdated drugs. She wanted to know more about mental health but the time left for clinical work, let alone for thinking of the patient within, was constrained. No, Rose insisted, being in charge gave a buzz, and motivated the two of them and she was committed to the practice as a result. She thrived on change and having responsibility. Yet being all things for many people could also distract from the main purpose.

A Poorly Performing Partner

Dr Saraswarthy (the name means female Goddess of wisdom and was chosen as a pseudonym by the doctor; 'Sara' for short) is deeply committed to working with diverse ethnic populations. She knew, as a refugee herself, what it meant to be dislocated and uprooted from your country. It was the final interview and Sara told me she wanted to take a risk and share a problem that was oppressing her. She was busily advising others on clinical governance and practice development plans. And yet she was deeply troubled by her own imperfections, feelings of failure and poor performance. She found it difficult to raise matters with GP colleagues for fear of being thought inadequate. Her case might be one from which others could learn.

She was in despair, she said, about a colleague and his performance. He was the kind of poorly performing doctor everyone complained about and with justification. Sara played a leading role in various professional development initiatives throughout the area and had facilitated a number of learning groups for single-handers. Yet she was stuck with a problem and her own anguish about performing badly in relation to it. 'People, colleagues, only know and see part of the picture,' she said.

The GPs' Responsibility

Sara insisted that GPs themselves had to take more responsibility for addressing the problems of poorly performing colleagues. General practice had to become a more transparent service, with a better-educated body of

GPs. They also needed to be accountable to patients and to the wider public in a new kind of social contract where each party knew their mutual responsibilities and rights. But Sara felt this should be done without undermining professional autonomy and morale. The desire to learn could be stifled by excessive surveillance and minimal trust.

She thought the morale of many doctors was on the edge. There was no funding, post-LIZEI, to tackle problems of underperformance and manage the changes required. She knew the problems, the people and their practices, more than most. Most doctors, she believed, were willing and able to change and learn if the process was managed humanely and the objectives and methods could be 'owned' by the GPs. But she was concerned about change being managed in hard and 'macho' ways. This made it difficult to face, openly, problems of underperformance, including in her practice. To be too open, when single-handers were under such attack from colleagues and bureaucrats, could be dangerous.

Personal Dimensions

The clinical performance and behaviour of her assistant gave her sleepless nights. Sara was shortly to face a medical hearing where he, the assistant, had made a complaint against her for denying him the opportunity to become a partner in the practice. She had wondered if this was the time 'to expose a colleague who is, in my opinion, underperforming'. The choice was hard and she wanted to consider the matter with me. 'This is a reality in primary care, which research should document, if it was to be of use,' she said. There was too much secrecy and she wanted to tell the story because: 'It is relevant – most practitioners have this problem.'

Psychological Problems

She had been concerned for a while about her colleague's clinical competence. He was a good human being but with psychological problems:

> He suddenly goes at a tangent and does a lot of things which are irrational. And sometimes he is very fine, very nice, accommodating ... To give an example, I advertised the post of partner and he was arguing with me about partnership and things and I asked him to apply for this partnership. So that in open forum he can appear and then be selected. I knew he wouldn't but I wanted to give him that option. He did not want to take it, so I got him to put it in writing to say that he doesn't want to do it. And I gave him a written statement saying that once a

person is selected I will give four weeks notice to leave. But on the day the interview was held, in the evening, he produced a memo, on a sticky pad, saying 'Thank you for keeping me for so long. I am very happy to leave in four weeks, once you have selected a person', and he dated it and handed it to me even without my letter saying that he should leave now that we have selected ... what went through his mind I don't know.

He, like her, was from a minority background and finding work, elsewhere, would be difficult. Sara had tried to manage the problems of underperformance, gently and developmentally, over a long period. There were 'many deviations' from what might be considered minimum standards but she had never 'had the heart or the courage to put it in writing to implicate him in this underperformance'. Sara thought of herself as a facilitator and educator, working developmentally to help colleagues in their learning. She knew the profession could be difficult and unfair for minority doctors. She convinced herself there was another way. There had been many opportunities to sack him and she could submit 'any number of cases' of poor clinical practice and erratic behaviour. She eventually compiled a dossier when matters deteriorated badly:

One thing he was breaching confidentiality. He was talking to patients about me. Patients have complained. I went back to the patients and got them to write down what was said and they have given me this in writing. And a child of nine months was given antibiotics and dioralyte and rehydration fluid and hyper antibiotics; even an ordinary person will know this is wrong. But he did that and then that night the mother rang me to say that this has happened and I trusted him and this is what happened. I got annoyed with how he had dealt with this child and I said 'Stop it straightaway', but the diarrhoea wouldn't stop because the antibiotics were causing the diarrhoea. The mother took the child to the hospital and the consultant was annoyed, the paediatrician, and the paediatrician has told him, 'Look this is the wrong thing to do', and the patient came back to us, to me.

... And the mother came back to me saying that this is the situation and that this is the wrong thing to do, so I collected all this information and put it before him and said, 'Look this is not right', and to that the reply was – 'Don't try to tell me, I have more experience than you have and this is not wrong.' And then I got a letter from him, afterwards, on a piece of sticky paper saying that he had been trained in such and such a place ... with so and so and that he has worked with surgeons, using bio surgery, antibiotics ...

Sara told him what had been done was dangerous. He would not accept this although he stopped issuing prescriptions for antibiotics. At that time, Sara said, she could and should have sacked him on the spot so she wondered why she had failed to act.

She was frightened, for one thing, of being taken to court by a man whom she experienced as paranoid and aggressive:

He is divorced and is paranoid. And I had this fear that he may take me and do all sorts of things. He was fearing me and I was fearing him ... I won't come into the room alone, I usually bring someone because I am so scared and he has told me he is so scared of me that when he sees my car parked he doesn't come in. He told me that as well. I feel sorry for him as well. Can you see that? Funny state of affairs ... The only thing I always point out is that there is nothing against him personally, it is about the quality of service. That is what I point out all the time. And so now you can see how if this is the case with an assistant who works with me, who I pay, now clinical governance is not going to be easy with my colleague over there, he is independent, he does his own thing. So how are you going to handle that? ... So this is an experience I have gone through where I now feel that I have failed in my duty to take the right procedures and get him seen by the GMC structure.

Sara had been dependent on him while she was establishing herself in the profession. She wanted the practice to be a beacon for what single-handers could do. She was working, at the time, on new audit procedures but she felt guilty that she might have neglected problems in her own practice, including her assistant:

'I am a coward, simple as that.' Yes. I didn't have the courage to say it. I despised him, not as a person, as a doctor. Yes well, in the sense that sometimes he may go berserk. He may start writing to ministers or he may start writing all sorts of things about me. And once it is open then how can I undo that? It is difficult. So I just carry on and hope that this goes away. Whether it was going through my mind in this order I don't know. Maybe all these factors came. It is more complicated than can be expressed ... But afterwards when I started, when I was clearly decided that I must get rid of him, then the conflict was between him taking me to a hearing, constructive dismissal, harassment etc., all these factors coming into play. All this, so I wanted slowly to slip him out somehow without appearing to be harassing him ... Yes, yes. And looking back, what went through my mind at that time was that I didn't want any hassle. Looking back I didn't want any hassle. And so I wanted to kill it.

I raised the issue of feeling, perhaps, an outsider in medicine:

That was working in my mind all the time. Although I had been thinking about it several times. Because by nature over the years I have always been on the side of the underdog and I just couldn't live with that type of betrayal, shall we say ... so I didn't want to be on the side of exposing a colleague who is underperforming but I thought I could work with him and get him to improve.

... I was reluctant to do anything about it. You see I grumble about it. I feel very unhappy about how things are and every day when I come I have some problem to deal with, a legacy he has left behind. And this was bothering me all the time, but I mean I was stupid in many ways, not dealing with it there and then, although I have this open culture here. What a funny state it is. And I believed in openness and everything and as far as I am concerned the case is very open, but when it came to dealing with him I didn't do it properly. So this is a lesson I have learnt, absolutely.

I wondered if she had feared putting her achievements at risk in a male world:

Possibly yes. Consciously or unconsciously it may have been working on me

... Very interesting analysis. Maybe there is some truth in what you are saying. Maybe I was trying to protect my reputation as a person where these problems don't exist.

... No I understand that, because we are talking in confidence I don't mind sharing these types of thoughts about it because maybe it was working in me. Maybe that is why I wasn't dealing with him the way I should have ... Maybe yes, I have to prove myself.

Sara felt that poorly performing doctors from minority backgrounds were letting themselves, and colleagues, down, by failing to address underperformance. She felt strongly about some of the hypocrisy, including her own, over standards. More colleagues should engage in lifelong learning but failed to do so. Yet being of a minority, and a woman, drove her to be better than other people, to outperform the insiders:

We do it ourselves and then prove these are the things that have got to be done and they will listen to you ... Just because we are the underdog and we are in a minority if you are going to keep on getting into a corner and start grumbling nothing will happen ... The people from poor circumstances, from poor backgrounds and disadvantaged positions who do well are people who are driven to do things. And I am a firm believer that you have to do it. No one is going to do it for you ... And as a woman ...

11
Ethnic Edges

... but it is only within the medical school that such remarks are, clearly unwittingly, tolerated. Racial stereotypes, too, are not uncommonly voiced aloud or indicated non-verbally, as when an officer of the Students' Union rubbed his nose with his forefinger to a Jew, or a rugby player spread his lips to indicate a black man. As an Asian woman student recounted that after a bout of kissing ... he told her, 'You'd be great if you weren't black ...

Simon Sinclair, *Making Doctors*

Sub-texts

The barely concealed sub-text in many reports on standards of care in the inner-city is that some of the worst doctors are Asian and single-handers. Their standards are often unfavourably contrasted with the 'avant-garde' practices down the road. This chapter considers some stories from a number of Asian single-handers, working in London and the Medway towns. Two of the doctors work in Chatham, an historically homogeneous working-class community built around the docks and other large employers until the closure of the main sources of employment (petro-chemical industries as well as the dockyard) in the early 1980s. Communities like the Medway, as with parts of inner-London, have become a focus of acute anxiety concerning patterns of social exclusion and long-term unemployment spanning generations, as well as poor and declining levels of health (Ward, 1995; Commission on Social Justice, 1994). Chatham and its hinterland are multi-cultural with a substantial Asian population living there. Optimism can be limited, and racism can thrive, in such marginal lands.

Many of the Asian doctors on the Medway are middle-aged men and due to retire within the next few years. Some of their colleagues, in the Medway, considered them resistant to change and poor in crucial areas of the work. Dr Pearl Jones worked in a group practice in the area:

... some of the stories I hear ... it is horrendous ... I feel they have missed the issue of team work, because the whole point of the Primary Care Groups is to work with the nurses, Social Services, Trusts and work as a team, not as a hierarchy ... Frightening really, what sort of service they [the patients] get ... and it tends to be very much the complaint that people don't listen, particularly from the women and it is mainly men, male doctors around. You know they will go with a female problem and they will get dismissed – oh you know it is women's problems. I can think of one patient who registered with us, who came first registration with a huge list of menopausal type of problems and she'd been having them for years. And so I said – 'Well did you not go to your doctor?' and she said 'He said – oh yes it is just something that women have to put up with', and wouldn't give her any investigations. When I teased out what was going on and did some investigations she had thyrotox-icosis and it was actually quite severe thyrotoxicosis and this had presumably been going on all these years, masked and complicated by the menopause at the same time, but clearly that woman should have been investigated years ago and was just dismissed as 'women's problems' and therefore didn't go back ... There was a doctor that was struck off ... A lot of the Asian patients were with him because he was the local doctor, he was Asian, and he used to give them all an iron injection every year, so if any of these ladies who came to him weren't very well, they just got their iron injection. He didn't check that they were anaemic ...

Pearl was concerned that for too long far too little had been done to improve matters. She was conscious of seeming racist, but there was no excuse for poor and inadequate services.

A Complex Tale

Dr Patel took over the practice in Chatham, in the late 1980s, from a doctor who had been struck off the medical register. There was chaos for a while but there was now a full-size list, a practice manager, a nurse and a receptionist. If the surgery was small and the area hard, this was no 'lock-up shop', either.

Dr Patel trained as a general surgeon before becoming a GP:

... Suddenly you are sort of dealing with things, which in the past used to be done by nurses and, you know, junior doctors and things like that, whereas I was in a higher position than them, but academically I think it gave me a kind of sudden release, as it were. It gave me more space to sort of reflect. I used to be very interested in literature and things like that. I started a course in mathematics. That's partly because I could suddenly look into these things I couldn't do when I was in hospitals. But the inability to deal with a problem comprehensively like in hospital ... and sometimes you feel ... yes, it is powerlessness plus occasionally, I suppose in surgery where you are doing things, you're using your hands, you can see the results in front of you. And one thing moves on to another, every week there is something happening, as it were, but not in general practice.

He joined an experiential group, and shared some anxieties:

... there are times when you are really ... should I say stressed up, or when it's there ... what's the word for it? When you are deep down in extreme anxiety. Yes, I speak to my wife but then I have to go through the emotions over and over again in myself. Another thing I do is to ring up a close friend, a GP. But then again you see, when I speak to them they always sort of give you the words that you want to hear, kind of thing, which I don't trust either ... the next thing to do is to read up about similar situations and presentations and hopefully, over a period of time ... I had the singular instance of an aneurism ... I discussed with a group because another GP had the similar situation where somebody dropped dead two days later. So it was like a common problem. But it was helpful. I think ultimately it was a sublimation within myself, but it all helped ... one has to resolve within oneself and that's justifying in a kind of way ... I have to come to the solution, it has to be within me, whether there are a hundred people, or two or three, or myself. The ultimate solution is within me, so I don't know whether it would make any difference being in a group practice or not.

Dr Patel was a very private man.

Middlemarch

He talked about a patient making a complaint:

There was this lady who, you know, fell for me, or whatever, and in the practice or consulting room, she suddenly started kissing me, and you know, that sort of thing, but I didn't know how to handle this ... so I didn't know what to do in this situation, where it was all mixed, and then at lunchtime I suddenly got the jitters, so I rang up my previous trainer, who is not far from here, and the first thing he said was 'Take her off the list!' Then I thought to myself, I can't do that, I mean somebody whom I know very well. Then I spoke to a chemist and he said 'Keep off ... ', yes he didn't say very much I think. I can't remember exactly what he said, but these are the people I speak to immediately when I get a problem, so to speak, including the advisers at the Medical Protection Service ... I used to be in consultation with one of their advisers there. He said 'Whatever you do don't take her off the list. Just let it cool off.' And I think that was the best advice I ever got, because she came back again and you know, it was sort of different, it was the weekend ... and subsequently I realised I learned to make the glass plane. I told you there was a glass plane ... I always put a plane in between me and my patients ...

He was reading Middlemarch at the time:

> ... the banker suddenly got found out about this fraud that he had committed and he was the most respectable ... and suddenly it struck a bell. And this is what I mean about connections that I make in life through other people ... I think the world I look at it is a world of ideas, you know. These are all floating around and we are all sort of making connections and there is a wider picture ... So it suddenly struck me, with this woman, I am like this banker who had got drawn into this affair, and here's my wife. What if she hears about it?

Dr Patel described himself as restless, in search of solutions and existential purpose. He searched for certainty in mathematics:

> then I found when I did do mathematics I suddenly found that even in mathematics there are many conclusions, deeper ambiguities; takes you into philosophy ... and I found even that is not the answer at all because of the mysticism I think. I touched on that in ... the inaccuracy in mathematics. Even there the ultimate solution wasn't there. You can do little exercises calculating something or other and giving a final answer but that's just an exercise in some kind of jugglery but it was the ultimate truth I was after. And I suddenly realised it doesn't exist there either; mathematics is such a vague subject in the end.
>
> ... It's just that, I think we are all thrashing round trying to find the reason for existence, but then again one does get a little satisfaction from achieving something right in front of your eyes, like for example you diagnose something, send them to hospital and it turns out to be such and such and the person is cured. Then you get the satisfaction. I think sometimes it is nice to have that sort of shallow, when I say shallow I don't mean ... that sort of satisfaction which we used to get in

general surgery like when someone comes in with abdominal pain, a little child, you do an appendicectomy and the child goes home in a week, which is the usual sort of scenario. That sort of completeness is not in general practice.

Dr Patel was feeling especially low when we met for the final time:

And patients get very aggressive and they want antibiotics. For me it is very inappropriate. In the end I give up and just give it and that I feel is a complete defeat, where I haven't been successful in convincing somebody or even planning a kind of management structure to both parties' satisfaction; I find it adds to your stress then. The helpless feeling. I must confess there are times, like this morning I had one or two, where perhaps I don't know, maybe it's subjective, sometimes I feel as though there is more of it now than before; more of the dissatisfaction, dissatisfied customers as it were.

He thought patients were getting more insistent, wanting quick cures, as if by magic. Sometimes he felt 'dumped on', like the failing parent dealing with demanding children. He was angry about how GPs were sometimes treated in the profession:

... a consultant paediatrician, I won't mention any names of course so it won't really matter, who rang me up and said 'There is this young girl who you've referred who has constipation and can we make a better policy that they shouldn't have any ... not pessaries ... what do you call them ... glycerin ... not to use suppositories on this particular child', and I said 'Fine.' But then I said this was a very difficult family and she said 'Oh, she's extremely nice, they are a very nice family, everything's fine.' And that was the end of that. But what she didn't realise is the husband and the mother, they come every week to see us. Now they don't really understand the profile, the family profile, the understanding. There was a lack of insight into the individual in terms of health, family relationships etc. and a misunderstanding of the use of the term 'difficult'. And they are nice people, it is nothing to do with that, but when I said, I did mention the word they were a fairly difficult family, but 'Oh no, they're not difficult, they are very nice, I've met the wife. She's wonderful and ...' What I am trying to say it makes you just want to give up.

Racism existed in medicine, yet he felt 'more able and intelligent' than many colleagues and it did not worry him, and he did not see this as defensive. His problem was bigger, to do with the uncertainty and irresolution at the heart of general practice. There was a long pause at the end of the final interview. The phone rang, and a patient needed urgent attention. The research had been helpful, he said, in offering space to think. It was not easy to find time to do so, or to be open in medicine. There was much pretence. He kept himself to himself and colleagues knew little of what he really thought.

A Proud Man

Dr Anwar Tendulker was born into the Rajput caste of Hindu Warriors. The men commanded respect in Indian culture and he was the child of an educated and wealthy family. Entering medicine was normal for someone like him:

> In India medicine is still regarded as a super speciality where you have respect, you have command, you have money if you want to earn, and the main thing was the respect and you were treated as this person who can heal things, who can ease your pain, who can give you comfort. So in some communities and if you worked in village settings you were treated as a god, as God, here is someone who takes your pain away, who gives you better life, who can cure things and therefore if you said anything that was taken for granted. They trusted you. And you had a very high image in the society.

Anwar explained that whilst medicine offered the best opportunities, status and security, this was changing as the medical profession became less prestigious and Asian children wanted more freedom to make their own choices.

His Training

He was aware, now, more so than at the time, of the shortcomings of his training. He was interested in mental health, for which he had had no training:

> In student days there is also very little teaching about that aspect. I think everybody was clinically orientated, but you believed in finding a disease, which you can treat. I can't remember any session which was spent on looking at the psychological aspect and treating the psychology of the person. I am not sure what was the situation here at that time, so many years ago, but we were totally clinically orientated. We were just taught about how you diagnose a disease and how you

treat. What disease has got on the human psychology was not taught, and I think I became aware of that after coming to this country and more so when I moved into general practice. Even when I worked here in hospital that was not the case. Since moving into general practice and starting to take part in training I became more and more aware of this. Now when we look at a patient, I always think of three things: the physical, social and psychological aspects. I use that as a coat-hanger in every consultation. And if I find there isn't a physical cause, then I would look for a social cause for her or him coming, and if not I would look for a psychological cause, and then you feel you have looked at the person in total. But I remember in my medical school days I don't think we had any input about that aspect and therefore you could see how inadequate, how incomplete, was the knowledge that we were gaining.

Part of the problem was that Asian people were brought up to believe that psychiatric or psychological illness was tantamount to madness. He had believed that too.

Between Worlds

Anwar sometimes wanted to go home:

I think because where you were born and brought up, you have some sort of that inner feeling that in that setting, towards the latter part of the life, you would be able to offer more. You will be more tranquil, you know, what you call calm feeling in you rather than rushing around from here to there. And the community feeling, the joint family feeling is still in existence there. Here I could end up in a nursing home. There I don't think that would happen, especially where I will be living. I would not have any problem with people looking after me. I would never be short of people with me. I would never feel lonely and certainly if you compare the high tech. medicine and all that, if there is a need you might not be able to get that quickly as you would get here living in other cities, but for mental peace I feel that that would be a place. I am not sure that I would stay there all the time, stay for say nine months a year, because the children would be here. But that's the feeling you have. And that's the community you have.

... So you never feel lonely and that is another reason why people don't feel that depressed and anxious. People will not go to anybody saying they are anxious, suffering from anxiety. I have never heard anybody saying that they suffer from anxiety ... Perhaps those people who work in cities, it is happening, but in the rural settings, village settings, it still is a very calm and very comfortable life.

Racism came to feature more prominently in the later part of the research:

It is for you to find a job and the only referee you have is this particular consultant who you did the attachment with and then you start to apply and competition is such that those people who have got experience, who have contacts, they always get good jobs. So you wait for a while and then you have to say – 'Look I can't, I have to get anything, whatever I can.' So while you wanted to do medicine you would apply for those specialities, like geriatrics, psychiatry, casualty, because you want to survive, you want to get time to see if you can get things sorted out. Before you are saying OK, you are packing your bag and going. So that is something, which causes a lot of problems towards these doctors for quite some time. And you get so unsettled ... You land up doing more work without any respect. And a lot of overseas doctors did for years and years. It could take anything up to two years before you got a reasonably good job in a good institution and by that time you are mentally not very happy and because you had left everything at home ... There were so many people looking for jobs and the feeling we were given was that if you had a local applicant you stood no chance at all. And if you went for better jobs then there would be more local applicants, anyway, so we didn't apply for these jobs, teaching jobs in good hospitals. You knew that you had no chance at all of getting into there.

... I think it is the fault of the perception that those who were trained abroad didn't have the same quality of education and I am sure, and I think everybody is feeling, those who were in my situation, felt that there was racism. Because you know unless you give an opportunity to someone you cannot assess whether they can progress on the same ladder at the same speed or not ... you are allowed to come in but these are the jobs you can do ... and the feeling you had that you were needed for the areas where local people won't go. You know valleys, remote places, rough areas, inner-cities and you could see, even in general practice, that these even now have mostly overseas doctors. Rough areas, bad areas ... And that could be the one reason, because that is the only place they could get a job.

Racism invaded the surgery:

There are times when I have been told by the girls that I have got a patient who wants to see only white doctors. It makes you feel 'Why?'

Patients would do the same thing again. The way they would address sometimes. 'That such and such doctor, not that doctor, not Dr Tendulker'. I don't think any of the locals would feel that Dr Tendulker must have been a white doctor because the name itself tells. But sometimes these comments are made. And even the staff. I had a member of staff here who was an Asian girl and the patients would treat her differently compared to the white girls. Children face the same thing from time to time. School friends make remarks about the colour of the country they have come from and the one thing that always keeps cropping up now if their friends are unhappy they say 'go back' and these things always make you feel 'Why should we be different? We decided to stay here, we are doing everything that we should be doing.' You are not on the dole, not taking any money without working and still there are times when you get this feeling that why somebody has to say 'go home'. This is my home. Why should I go home? Why should I say that that is my home now?

... I remember one patient who came ... at the reception requesting some medications, repeat prescription. He is an alcoholic and whenever he came he always was under the influence of alcohol and always demanded 'I need this done now.' And most other times the receptionists would do this because they were scared that if he did not get it he would get violent and abusive. One day I was in the surgery when he became very rude and aggressive to the staff so they contacted me on the phone. And I decided to see him, and talk to him, that this is not the way to use the service and he agreed to come to my room. I offered him a seat and his response was that – 'Don't you ask me sit down, you don't know who I am. This is not your country, you are here to do what we are telling you to do.' And remarks like this, which was not necessary. And obviously I did not like this and still I did my duty to explain to him that 'What we are doing here is for yourself and it is for you to use the service properly so that everybody can benefit by that and the system is this', and he was not prepared to listen to me and he made several racist remarks. Then he walked out saying, 'I will get my son and he will sort you out.' And then when he walked out of the room his final remark was – 'Fuck off you, go back to your country.' I know that he did that because he was under the influence of alcohol, but it must have been in his mind, in his heart to be able to say these things to me when there was no argument with me ... When he went out to the reception he started to make racist remarks and was abusive and we had to contact the police to come and remove him ... I had an Asian girl at reception and people were unhappy. There were one or two occasions when they would not say anything to white staff, but she would get occasional remarks, which made her very uncomfortable at times and finally she left because she could not cope with this ... 'You are a Paki, what do you know about this country?'

There was particular poignancy in being treated this way:

> ... abused when seeking to care, of being sworn at when trying to help. The context was important when considering many Asian doctors ... some of these doctors, those who landed up in practices that were not taken up by other people. You know they were so choosy, they got other places, so Asian doctors, a lot of them, landed up in places that were not well equipped, had their own problems, you know, whether it is teenage problems, or drug addicts or too many elderly. There are problems like that. And we have poor working conditions. So obviously your performance is not exactly the same and we did work in single-handed practices that made life a bit difficult, because you need time to go out and attend courses and, you know, have some practice-based education which is difficult to organise for one person.
>
> ... There are no statistics to prove that their patients are less well looked after. There is no more morbidity and mortality, nobody has shown me. I have not read anywhere any statistics saying that they are underperforming ... They might be underperforming but if you talk about the premises and all that, staffing, the attitude of the Health Authority is not exactly the same way. If other single doctors go for extra staffing, invariably they are turned down. If you have got bigger practices and more powerful doctors you stand more chance of getting help financially staff-wise or IT-wise. So I don't think it is only the Asian doctors. I feel very strongly about it. And you know if you are powerful, if you are in group practices, you stand a good chance of getting further help. Single-handed doctors have been isolated. They have been left by the Health Authorities and agencies who should be supporting them.

Colleagues like him felt marginalised. Scapegoating single-handers was an exercise in avoidance. 'Medicine and medics heal thyself and culture', he said with feeling.

Diasporas

Dr Bedi was the product of the diaspora, the dispersal of the peoples of the former British Empire. This, as Stuart Hall (1992) has written, is the shared history of formerly colonised peoples moving to this country. It is a story of family fractures and subsequent attempts at recombination as well as assimilation. Dr Bedi's parents were born in India, while he was a product of East Africa and the fierce inter-racial strife that was the legacy of Empire. He had been in his present practice for about eight years, starting from scratch. He mentioned 'colour discrimination' early on and the fact that the practice in which he worked was born out of sheer frustration at not being able to find any other job in medicine in the United Kingdom.

He never intended to be a general practitioner and his first love was paediatrics.

> ... I loved children ... you see, and the paediatric ward, it was a very rewarding thing ... a child had come very ill and you are doing your three-monthly job in paediatrics. You left a child thinking 'Oh my God, I hope he is alive tomorrow.' And the next day you go onto the ward and the child is sitting up and drinking, eating and it is a matter of joy you see. And I thought that was very rewarding and nice. That is why I was paediatric-oriented and luckily enough my first job, I had to take up the first job that was available in the hospital and that was in paediatrics. Very fine job, because unlike here when I tell people they hardly believe it, we would have at least eight to ten deaths. We had two wards, sixty beds each and would have about ten or twelve, or fourteen, deaths ... Oh my God, initially it was very depressing. At times I was blaming myself. Was I doing enough? And one of my senior friends was there, he said, 'Bedi you are here. All that you can do is your best. Look at their records, the death rate there before you came in, so don't blame yourself. You are trying your best. You have got the help of your registrar, he comes on the ward, but these are very ill children coming. So what you can do is only your best.' ... We used to call it 'straw' syndrome. The professor used to describe it as straw syndrome. This child is only hanging by a straw, could have malnutrition, could have malaria, worms, pneumonia and gastro-enteritis, things like that. Dehydration. Kwasicor was our biggest problem, malnutrition, it looked like a well-nourished child but it wasn't. It looked well, but it wasn't. It was built-in calorie malnutrition and at that time tuberculosis was rampant.

The work was abandoned as the country and politics turned sour. He came to England but it was impossible for someone like him to get a post in paediatrics here. Life, in the meantime, was desperate at home and it was imperative to get his children out of Africa as quickly as possible. Being your own boss, and thus in control, was important:

Freedom to practice yourself and nobody is your boss ... I took up a temporary job in East Africa when I first went into employment. My father got me a job in the Government, a clerical job, and unfortunately I had a boss from South Africa and he didn't like me, I think, the colour of my skin and he irritated me once. He irritated me. He called me in his office and I leaned my hands on his table and he said 'Whoosh, hands off the table.' I felt a bit hurt. I went back and spoke to my colleagues where I was working, and they said 'This is what you will get. Can't do anything about it.' And I said – 'What do you mean you can't do anything about it? Can't treat people like this.' In about two weeks he was leaning his back on my table and I pushed ink on his pants and said, 'Whoosh, don't you lean on my table.'

But security was always fragile and involved keeping your mouth shut. The African was third class. Cricket was a metaphor for the whole system; the whites had a bat each, the Asians three between them while the blacks were lucky to have any at all:

It does shape me, and at times you see, you can become paranoid about it ... my first experience here was – I did my training job and then made about eighty applications, no replies. Then you start thinking, what is it? Is it you? Your degrees? I trained at the best college in India ... at that time it was the best college. I trained as a registrar ... with different consultants from America, Great Ormond Street, from England, Australia and I came and trained here in London. I got my Diploma in Child Health at the first shot, OK lucky, but I got it. I had done enough work in paediatrics to get it. And then when I don't get a job I start thinking and I used to tell my wife – 'Let's go back.'

... And my wife said no. And in those days when this independence thing was going on my father used to say something – 'When things are not going your way, stop blaming others. Put yourself up. Fight it you will get it.' And I started this practice ...

By and large he felt accepted by most patients. The problems had to do with poorly performing doctors and racism:

When I worked in a children's hospital we had several visiting consultants and the way they supported my application, each one of them recommended me for the job that I was looking for in paediatrics. An Australian got it and he did not have a Diploma in Child Health, whereas I had already acquired a Diploma in Paediatrics. That disappointed me a bit. I went and spoke to my boss and he said that he could not help me there because it involved several people – all had to be consulted and they opted for the other candidate ... twenty or twenty-five years ago the only jobs that coloureds got were in geriatrics or psychiatry or anaesthetics. Top jobs in general surgery or medicine, neurology was a difficult one unless you were an exceptionally brilliant person, which I think I wasn't ...

He found it harder to raise such issues then, and felt it was not the done thing to ask too many questions.

We spent most of the final interview considering present changes in the role of the GP. He disliked the 1990 contract, which he thought had been imposed upon doctors, but had tried to make it work. Fundholding offered some opportunity for control:

Immediately I realised that it was a sort of two-pronged practice, the fundholders who had a free hand to do whatever they wanted to do, I made attempts to get into fundholding, but then came this little news again that they were going to squeeze the budgets to such an extent that even the new fundholders were not very happy and it looked like you see they are going to be changing Government and fundholding will go ... And I knew one day it will disappear. It can't go on. But I am now totally having mixed feelings as to the direction we are going.

He mourned the passing of the family doctor:

That you are a doctor to the entire family and you knew each one of them ... Because society is changing now isn't it? When you talk about a family practice, you are talking about ten or fifteen families that I have, where thirty or forty members of the family are in my practice and I know them as a family.

As for the criticisms of Asian single-handers:

... Nonsense. Speaking from my practice ... At the end of the day ask the recipient, the patient, and by and large, not because I am a single-handed practitioner, by and large when you talk to people they say when I go to that surgery now, I see the same GP. I am not a number. It becomes very easy for a general practitioner to know all his patients. When you are in a group practice I think you become a number. They are quite happy. I do not see why single-handed practitioners should be underperforming ... I think it totally wrong to say that they are under-performing ... OK, if there is anything that we are not doing and you expect us to do, let us know, but respect the single-handed practitioner because he is delivering far better goods and I can assure you that we are delivering far better goods than group practices are doing. This practice achieves every criterion that is set in, say, immunisation, cervical cytology. My home deliveries, although I am single-handed, whether I do the home deliveries is another issue, but as long as the women have that freedom and they are going to have a home delivery, I do home deliveries. So where are we going to underperform?

But he recognized there were problems, due to changing roles. Treatments were different now and a doctor needed to keep up to date. Group practices were at an advantage there since GPs could take time off to do a course, which was not easy for a single-hander.

So the role of a general practitioner has changed. The general practice role has now become more of administrating ... For instance if my patient has any surgery, by-pass surgery being done, he is going to be back home after seven days you see. And his care is going to involve myself as a GP, my practice nurse, or district nurse, and the other Social Services Department. There are implications because of his by-pass surgery, and I think the general practice nurse has to become a sort of a kingpin to make sure that all this happens. That role has changed now, hasn't it? The practice load and work has changed you see and I see two kinds of role that I am here. I am the GP there to look at sore throats, coughs, colds. I know exactly when they walk in and what they are going to get out with. Advice, a little Calpol, go home and come back, but the other role has changed because the pattern of practice has changed ... I didn't know anything about HRT, neither did I bother ten or fifteen years ago. HRT. I have got to know about HRT, depression, and the amount of depression and things that we are facing today that we ought to know practically as much as the consultant psychiatrist knows you see ... If ever we are going to reduce suicides and we are going to reduce people suffering from depression ... Here in general practice, we have got to look out and that is where the role has changed. I think those days are gone when you could say OK I am going to have fifteen appointments.

He was nearing retirement, felt tired and sometimes sad about present trends. It was time to finish.

Another Sadness

John Chandra's family were Brahmins, the priests of the caste system. Brahmins were not supposed to touch excreta or sputum ... but his father, who was a doctor, went his own way. John came to England in the 1960s:

... I didn't get the jobs, I was lined up for a surgical registrar job, which I did not get. So it was a big disappointment at the time because to work in that hospital and to be a senior registrar means you could walk into any hospitals of the world at the end of it. But strangely enough, it was not a big setback for me ... it shattered me but I cannot recall being depressed because I did not get it ... I am surprised why I was not depressed. I should have been in an asylum after that because though I was given an alternative surgical registrar, but comparing that to what I was going to get, and for the sacrifice I had to leave my wife for nearly eight years.

Racism was quite acceptable in those days because doctors from the Indian sub-continent did not aspire to achieve the same as their white counterparts. They knew their place.

Psychological Medicine

John had been in a Balint Group for two years but still felt inadequate in relation to mental health issues. There was a patient, for instance, in the surgery that morning:

... This is a lady in her sixties who kept coming with complaints which were not necessarily trivial, but which needed attention, like loss of appetite, abdomen pain, even going on to the extent of investigating and finding something positive like gall stones. Now one could panic, 'Oh well we have found something, we will get it treated and that will be the end of it.' But since I had a surgical background I was quite happy to handle that this is a gall bladder, which doesn't need an operation. Just to say it briefly if it is a single gall stone it is usually a metabolic stone, they don't need treatment necessarily, but if there are multi-gall stones and they are infective they need to have the gall bladder out. So I was capable of handling that and I didn't refer her to a specialist but I referred in a way as I did lots and lots of investigations to make sure that she was all right. And then it came up that she is rather lonely, she has lost most of the members of her side of the family and her husband was a little bit indifferent. She had been moving her house from one council house to the other, for something like ten years.
... The issues raised were not to jump on to the prescription pad and write 'anti-depressant' at the first sight of seeing a patient who is down. Be brave and do the counselling even in the areas where you feel inefficient, like homosexuality, or relationship problems, having had no

experience, but be brave and listen. I learned that listening is a therapy in itself.

There were boundary problems:

> And one day, one evening, she came and we talked and this went beyond the time of closure of the surgery, to the extent that I forgot to pick up my daughter from school. I was supposed to, and that was a very uncomfortable evening because I said, 'Oh I must leave you now, I was supposed to pick up my daughter from school', and I rang my home immediately and asked my wife if Irinda had come, and she said 'No she hasn't, we were wondering where you were.' I said 'I am still in the surgery.' So I went to the school, obviously she had left and she went to the bus stop. I picked her up from the bus stand and I shared that with the Balint and they said 'You are concerned that you want to help this woman. This woman is challenging, her husband is extremely demanding and sometimes threatening to you, you know.' ... Yes I felt sucked into her problem ...

John felt his life was unbalanced at times. He was working harder, to the neglect of his family. He still needed to prove himself and worked overly long hours to do so. Sometimes he felt 'slightly backward in the sense that you don't know what is going on around you'.

Single-handers

The treatment of single-handers upset him:

> ... single-handed practitioners are step-motherly treated by the Health Authorities and I think they are lying by saying that prescribing costs are higher for single-handed GPs. I think they are also lying by saying that single-handed GPs are not performing too well. Because both things are incorrect. They think of drug-saving incentives and ever since it has been introduced, I have been in receipt of the incentive two years in a row, and I don't think I am an exception to other single-handed GPs, but what is happening now with the changing environment in the NHS as a whole, fundholding made a lot of savings and the Government went on the bandwagon and are going for a super fundholding like PCG now, and what the Health Authorities are looking at is saving, not the patient care, the savings, savings by being in one building, savings by using resources effectively. It may be true, but I am not too sure it is true ... A bit like a salaried GP now, because this is what the Health Service is doing. So I feel saddened really because the Health Service is

destroying the traditional general practice. I think, and I am not saying because I am single-handed, and I want to, I am single-handed, but I am also saying because I know the virtues of being single-handed, and not necessarily the disadvantages of it. I can see in ten years time the NHS will disappear. I hope it doesn't, but it may disappear. But by that time I will have retired.

He too was feeling low at our final interview. He looked out of the surgery window:

But yes there are occasions when you come against hurdles. That was one of the hurdles ... but it is all money-driven and if you happen to be of ethnic origin you do not get the same privileges that many others will get and my situation is one of these examples. Just to elaborate, since you asked me, we were granted an extension, only up to the trees some six years ago and the Health Authority knew the potential of this practice and my personal potentiality. They know that I am capable of doing lots of things. They want me to have larger premises and to have partners and even have a salaried partner from the Health Authority working in the premises. But because of what I am maybe, it could be more than being of ethnic origin, it could even be my age, they are thinking 'Is it worth investing in a man like him who has worked very hard all his life and might leave?'

He was counting the days, he said, until retirement. There was no role for him in the local PCG either. He had hoped to take the lead in clinical governance, but it was not to be. He shook his head and smiled a sad smile, 'Time to get on, Linden.'

Threads

These were stories of careers blighted in a medical world where racism has been persistent and hopelessly muddled with questions about standards; or career progress has depended on who you know in a white as well as a male world. A healthier profession would, it is suggested, place more value on diversity and on addressing the misogyny and racism in its ranks (Sinclair, 1997). The real issue, as Richard Schmitz (1996) has observed, might have to do with how people treat each other. Human beings are intrinsically social and relationships with others are the means to being more human. What is central to genuinely human relationships, and to learning about self, is to perceive difference as a means to growth and understanding, rather than a threat.

No doubt the stories above can be dismissed as unrepresentative and partial. Yet they represent real perceptions and deeply felt truths that matter for the health of the whole profession. Some doctors have felt abused, isolated, and unsupported; and it is hard to learn in such circumstances. Some have fought back and damaged their health in the process. But a growing number might be realising that their experience says as much, if not more, about the health of medicine, as it does about them and their performance.

12
Man to Man

> ... Traditional 'masculinity' focuses on dominance and independence, an orientation to the world which is active and assertive, which valorises competitiveness and turns its face from intimacy, achieving esteem in the glorification of force. The fear at the heart of this image is of emotion – that which makes us vulnerable and 'womanly'; emotion is dangerous not only because it implies dependence, but also because it is alien ... Representative of all that masculinity rejects.
>
> D. Glaser and S. Frosh, *Child Sexual Abuse*

Masculinity and Story

If the doctor's role is being questioned so, too, are some dominant fictions of masculinity, albeit on the margins. This penultimate chapter is the story of a successful 'public' man who yet, over time, anguished about the personal and emotional price paid. David Levine used the research to take stock and reconsider what was core, and what peripheral, to the work. Moreover, our relationship changed; at first this was formal while the story of being a doctor was a very public narrative, it then developed and evolved into a collaborative exploration of being a doctor, and men, in the present moment. David is a socially progressive doctor, who questions inequalities in health and the disparity in resources between the peoples of the inner-city and those of leafy suburbs and shires. He is angry at the neglect of the East End and, like David Widgery, with the politics of individualism and the minimalist state. The story might have ended there, but we were able to share narratives at a more intimate level too, and to connect public and private men, one life history with another.

A Successful Public Man

David Levine, on his own admission, presents the image of a confident, assured doctor, a 'politico' who knows the ropes:

I am constantly involved with changes, at least at one edge of general practice ... so I am meeting a lot of GPs and thinking a lot with other people about what the Health Service is for, what it is going to be like and what the general practitioner's role will be in that ... Just that there is a White Paper coming out tomorrow which will set the future of the NHS for the next ten years, but it is going to be a mixture of good and bad, but I am very worried that it is going to be very bad. I am personally quite agitated and anxious about it. I shall be glad when I know what it says and I think that what I am observing about general practice is, on the one hand a break-up of the monolith; there are going to be different ways of being GPs in the future, which I actually applaud. But, as so often, it is this worry of throwing away the good things with some of the bad. So it is the whole issue, for instance, of what it means to be a family physician rather than a general practitioner, and I think there is a difference.

David had mixed views about the health of general practice. Many doctors did well, against the odds, but, overall, the record was poor in the neglect of a public health strategy and in working multi-professionally. We talked about *A Fortunate Man*, and the idea of the GP as clerk to the family records. Continuity of care was important but doctors like John Sassall lacked a wider political perspective. Sassall thought that if he worked harder, and was nicer, and gave more to each patient, it would get better. Of course it did not; there are bigger socio-structural issues than that, shaping people's lives and well-being.

David stated that 'GPs were often their own worst enemies.' Bad practice had never been properly addressed, in the name of maintaining an independent profession. GPs had resisted standard setting, peer review, or being managed at all. Some practices and practitioners were very bad, '... there is always a huge gradient between people that are heavily involved [in education] and those that aren't'. Change was required urgently; the big issue was how to manage it and on what terms.

Contradictions

David thought this to be a contradictory moment with a conflict at the heart of the new Labour government between being NHS-friendly while zealously controlling public expenditure. Some proposals could even exacerbate the worst 'GP elitism':

And here we are on the eve of the White Paper and I don't know but I fear that they will be doing some market-type things to the Health

Service and they will be putting false power in the hands of people like GPs, so the threats of GPs holding a budget, albeit collectively, 90 per cent of the budget for health care for 100,000 population is just an awful prospect. I actually think it is untenable and it's not quite what we are going to find tomorrow, but we might. So where should the power lie? Power should be shared but it should be shared between the people that have responsibility in an area, so that is Health Authorities, Trusts and GPs, along with Social Services, but we are a long way from achieving the three, let alone bringing social care in. That is where it should be and power should be with people being able to access decent services, although I understand there have to be people involved in taking decisions and planning.

There was a new and healthier emphasis on 'pro-activity' and setting targets for practices and primary care. Targets were a good idea, the question was 'which targets' as well as how they were measured. This was something many GPs said they wanted and could influence if they chose to. The three partners in his practice were enthusiastic about present possibilities; of being able to manage themselves more effectively, and in a planned way, which could mean meeting a range of specified needs while also targeting resources on the people who most needed them.

Healthy relationships between professionals were crucial, but this was against a backcloth of rivalries and medical elitism. David's long-term solution involved radical changes to initial professional training, including agreeing objectives for primary care as a whole, as a first step, nationally, and then deciding how to train people to become team players. At present, people were trained in 'twenty different ways and then expected to work as a team':

And I think that the issue is that primary care and general practice have been bowling along for a hundred years and all of a sudden someone has turned the spotlight on them, which is what has happened since the early Nineties and we have yet to begin, well we are now beginning, to ask the right questions about how you organise primary care and how you manage it, in its broadest sense. How you set some sort of objectives for it and therefore how you can commission for it. We are only just at the beginning of that even though we have had the spotlight since 1990. So for me it's a mixture of good and bad news. The good news is that they have discovered us, even though we have been here for God knows how long, and the bad news is that they are getting some of it wrong in addressing the issues because they have no experience and by they I mean officials in the Government, NHS

Executives, regional people, local Health Authority, because there isn't the experience in there to understand how you do it. Nobody has really set about the task of planning the delivery, never mind the commissioning, of primary care.

Many health service managers were rigid and old-fashioned, hierarchical and prescriptive, rather than facilitative and empowering. This worried him deeply and was a major obstacle to progress. The rhetoric of collaboration in health care was often strong but the reality weak. Fundholding had addressed certain problems, including the inertia that could bedevil general practice, although it was never designed to this end but rather to save money. However, non-fundholding practices had been left behind in the development stakes:

> ... Well, we have a marvellous machine potentially at someone's disposal, which is in touch with the community, which had a national system of notes that are lifelong with the patient. We are developing a national patient number and we have IT on the desks of most practices. We have the capacity to do what we want, the question is what do we want to do? And it should be possible to target either in terms of current prescribing and looking at current prescribing in an imaginative way and saying, 'How are we going to manage this and what is good and what is bad and what works and what doesn't?', rather than relying on random control trials in hospitals. And similarly for targeting 'hard to reach' groups because poverty is one of the biggest determinants of health ... we should have advice workers in the practice ... for people we know are likely to be ill, but we don't get to, suffering from blood pressure and diabetes and heart disease. So there doesn't seem to be a difference between a proactive general practice and a public health view of what we should be doing. It's a very broad view and that fits completely with being able to commission from the primary care perspective because the needs presented to you are pretty clear. It is just a question of collecting it and then developing the plans to meet the needs coupled to available resources.

A research and development agenda could solve, in part, the problems of burn-out and poor morale among many doctors, allowing those with experience to engage more systematically in researching and developing general practice. Collective wisdom could be imaginatively harnessed:

> You have got to get to people before then, so that you don't get grumpy old men of fifty seeing lots of patients. Because that's going to be no

good at all. So there is a way in which this development can either be visionary – getting people to open out as they get older and more experienced – or it can actually be a disaster where you have to grind yourself into the dust before you earn the right to do something else, which is actually how consultant jobs work.

Medical Training

Medical training was a mess, David said, 'a process of selective brain damage'. It was noticeable, he thought, that in the year GP registrars might spend in a practice, they would often get depressed after six months. A good training would enable them to use a follow-up period to refocus their abilities:

> You don't cure patients. You may help them with the symptom, but they keep coming back because they are on your list. For me personally I have never had a model of medicine in my head that meant I was going to do anything particularly useful with it, to be honest. I see it as incredibly limited and the most powerful bit of my armament, if you like, is my ability to communicate with people, far more important in some respects, leaving aside who has had a heart attack, a defined medical problem, but in terms of being a day-to-day GP the most important thing I offer is the ability to sit and listen and reflect. That is the job. So I have never had the concern, in fact quite the opposite, I was very, very critical of my own training at the time it was going on. That was easy because it was in the Sixties and early Seventies when there was quite a lot of student activity going on. And we were questioning what we were told. So I have never had the problem of thinking that medicine is up to much. And I think it often does more harm than good, particularly if you let loose people like me who don't have the reflective side which can turn into being quite penalising towards patients. An obvious example is – 'Why won't you lose weight? Unless you do you will have a heart attack'. 'There I told you so.' Smoking behaviour, booze, whatever. And instead of being able to live with the patients at the level at which they experience life, you just become patronising, and judgemental and ultimately alienated from the job.

Personal Affairs

There was, we were later to agree, a formality and stiffness in our conversation. The private side of David was kept under wraps. Two years into the study, the story evolved, partly because he felt tired of the politics, partly because we got know each other better:

Yes, manoeuvring, political manoeuvring, small people, political manoeuvring which I have never been interested in and is just showing people in a bad light – I haven't enjoyed it and am glad I am out of it really ... there is a sort of sense of feeling aggrieved and put down, which I am grappling with, but it is linked in with some difficulties I am facing outside the practice in my own life that have nothing to do with that sort of area. And the feeling that although the NHS is moving on with the right principles, this is a very right-wing Labour Government who are probably either going to out-manoeuvre people, so that the principles seem to remain, but the implementation is awful, or else they might just chuck a load of money at the NHS in order for the NHS to be its star in the banner when it goes to the next election. But that will be at the cost of education, housing, tax on poverty and all the rest of it, so I am not satisfied with the Labour Government that we have got or how they are going to implement their policies.

A number of the Asian doctors had been targeted, as David put it, for 'special attention' over clinical standards. Their reaction was to organise themselves politically to defend their interests. Many were feeling vulnerable, and had attacked him for betraying their interests in meetings with the Health Service. This distressed him, although he understood why they were behaving as they were. Rather than praising Asian doctors for managing in difficult contexts, many were being pilloried; a blaming and scapegoat culture had long been in existence.

He was depressed, moreover, by what he perceived to be creeping privatisation. Primary care and general practice faced pressure on budgets and this could mean that drug companies would be asked to put more money into the NHS, enabling them to sell their drugs via so-called 'managed care packages'. This could be primary care's version of the Private Finance Initiative in hospitals. The Government was creating a virtual NHS, 'the one it thinks it is producing and is trying to sell to the public, and the real NHS is in chronic crisis':

... The bad side is to start setting GPs up to fail, rather like they have set teachers up to fail, to produce league tables, which say – 'this is good, this is bad', and without any account of how hard you actually have to work to achieve whatever you achieve, and setting people up to fail as knocking their confidence as professionals, saying to them, 'You are going to have to get reaccredited as a professional. You are going to have to meet certain quality standards. We are going to be sending people round to investigate you, your practice, or your Primary Care Group if we think you are not working properly', and all that is brand new and that can be quite punitive and unpleasant. And the example that I would give is the experience we had over Tomlinson, when someone had the bright idea of getting bad GPs to retire and of giving them £100,000 handshake and each Health Authority was asked to prepare a list of GPs that they would recommend for this immediate retirement package. And what they did was they looked at the only available data they had, which was some of the information they had about smears and immunisations, and the all the rest of it, and they therefore used their own local knowledge and prepared a hit list. So there is a way in which these things can be subverted, and people come out with appalling opinions about who is a good or a bad professional ... So there is a bad side to the Government's glitz actually resulting in a non-reflective look, and a poor judgement made about where the money should go and how it should be used ... The issue is what do you do, and again the Tomlinson example shows that what governments, what managers tend to do is they look round for someone to blame. So they blamed the influx of Asian doctors that arrived here in the Fifties and Sixties for the poor performance of inner-city general practice. Whereas actually what they should have done is congratulated them for having stuck it for thirty years with no resources, no one giving a damn about them. So it is seeing what actually is the problem and framing the problem correctly. Having framed the problem correctly then you know a variety of solutions begin to appear, and again the Tomlinson experience showed that, when there were people around to say to the NHS 'No, it is not about blaming people, it is about providing them with some head space to do all the things we need.' We are back to education, back to some of the initiatives that took place under Tomlinson and they succeeded.

David was soon to be fifty-five:

Depression probably applies to my own private life as well. And therefore a time to sort of lick my wounds, re-evaluate. I am fifty-five this year and hopefully will emerge after the summer feeling 'I know where I am going. I know what I am doing and I am enjoying building the practice up again.' Working with partners, or whatever ... Only that the difficulty I am facing personally has coincided with the changes I have just described and it is sometimes quite difficult to disentangle or see them separately, and if you get down, are you getting down because of what is happening in the personal and private, and you have just got to try and keep a clear head about which belongs where. But it is difficult; when you have been pushing at a door and it opens you can fall flat on your face. And to a certain extent, emotionally, I have, although I predicted I would. So there is the sort of regeneration of my own libido going on as well.

... I do experience a problem of coping with the level of stress and demand and expectation on me and to do it day in and day out for a large number of years obviously takes its toll. For me the politics is not so much my escape as it is my anti-depressant. If I am fighting I don't get depressed. I get depressed when I am confused, when I don't know which way to strike out, when I don't know how to deal with whatever is oppressing me. Once I have discovered that then I become less depressed.

... I have always felt an outsider and not accepted the given, always ... It is quite difficult for me to feel at ease with a bunch of doctors at a meeting on educational grounds, because the assumptions that are underlying the process of education are often incredibly different. So during my own year as a registrar when I was in a fairly typical sort of training, I was coming into conflict all the time with the assumptions, whether they be political assumptions, you know assumptions about racism, you know shared racism, you know shared sexism, shared patient bashing. They are all things that doctors assume that other doctors immediately share. And I don't.

Clinical work was taking its toll:

... There is no doubt about that. And I get ratty, angry, fed up. I still have the experience of sailing through a surgery and then one event will upset me and I will find it quite difficult to get myself together and try not to be a pig to the next five people. Constant monitoring battle. It is the third eye that you have to develop, monitoring and watching your own behaviour. And there are strategies. I will sometimes stop for five minutes, however busy it is. I will stop. I walk and get patients, call them personally because that walk through the office rehumanises me, or de-isolates me, or does something. Even though it is a pain when people ask you three different things. But at least it is interacting again. So all those sorts of things are coping strategies and are terribly important. But the fundamental one is to ask myself how I would react in their position. If someone is downright rude and a pig and got a mobile phone in one hand and the Patients' Charter in the other, I will actually do whatever the medical bit is and then actually pull them up. If I think they are abusing me, or the system, or the receptionists or whatever. We all have a commitment to do that. We are not here to be shat upon just because we are here.

There was a good argument, he said, for salaried GPs. There was abundant evidence that GPs were under-earning as well as under-achieving in difficult social areas, and being overwhelmed by the scale and complexity of the work. Having to be an employer and manager as well as a clinician was asking too much:

> Why are we all spending so much time employing half a dozen recep-tionists and secretaries where it would be more sensible for the area to do it once? So that is another reason. But it also puts you inside a framework when you are employed. You are actually expected to be inside a management structure. So it opens the door to time off for education, time off for sickness, time off for parenting, time off for, whatever, anyway, in the contract.

Yet David also recognised a conundrum, in that management in the NHS was frequently punitive and unimaginative while trust, rather than Trusts, was in scarce supply.

Diversity

David talked more about his family, and I about mine, and my history of political involvement and disillusion. I had been a 'politico', too, and there was also, in my case, a dissonance between the personal and public in my life. I was a child of the 1960s, wanting to build the new and better world, and believed the focus on the subjective was indulgent and irrelevant to action. Men like me called for the new society, but forgot that the women were making the tea (West, 1999). Action, for me, also disguised some deep personal insecurity and a need to perform to earn others' praise. The emotional was a place to be avoided because it was threatening to the public man (West, 1996). We began to share stories.

David talked too of his personal life:

> ... It is possible to analyse things in terms of coming home, in the sense that I have been absent from there more than I should have been, and it is an open discussion with myself and my wife that she acknowledged that (a) I was doing something that she supported but also (b) it left her without me, and without even when I was there – my head was elsewhere, and I have said many times and probably said it to you that without her particular support it would have been impossible. If there had been a background of rows and resentment it would have been utterly impossible for me to have devoted the time and attention, and it is time and attention, to what I did. So the end of the campaigning

and the change in what is going on, and the transitions that we have talked about have enabled me to go home as well. So I have had more time doing nothing at home in the last two months than I have done in the last eight years. So yes, dramatic, in a sense ... I mean as an individual I am constantly going through cycles of re-evaluation and looking and thinking about whether what I am doing is what I should be doing, want to be doing, all the rest of it. I received an Email from a friend who for all sorts of reasons just wrote to me and he said – 'David, what are you doing about yourself? Never mind about everything else.' Because I used the phrase, I used the phrase that working is my anti-depressant ... And I used it to him obviously as well and he wrote back and said 'Yes, but actually have you thought about pleasure?' And it is not a new idea to me but the concept that comes to me, and it might be a defence, but it feels sort of more or less right, is that for me to integrate my work, my political ideas and my home into a whole so that there is actually not a lot of difference between any of those is an integrated person to me. Others looking may say 'Well how come you know his home life consists of deep and meaningful chats with his wife, deep and meaningful chats with endless people on the phone, hitting the word processor, having a heavy job and that is what his life is.' And I am saying well that is actually fine. You could say to me, 'Yes but what about music, what about going to art, what about socialising?' and yes, yes, yes, that is all possible, but to be honest and frank I don't terribly much enjoy socialising with people who don't have that as a sort of given, because it is a bit pointless. I am not, I don't want to convert individual middle-class GPs, or their families, or similar people ... but I don't want actually to knock my head at a brick wall ... I mean I would like to get back to playing music. I would like to get back to, to having once a fortnight, once a week, actually going out and having a meal and a chat with people that I want to. And yes that is sort of on the cards. My wife has been ill ...

Her background was different from his:

... Mary has always had difficulties, emotional of one sort or another, and to do with her experience of being a woman and to do with her experience of coming from quite a deprived family, but that had never got resolved and she had a crack-up some years ago and has now been depressed for a couple of years and is now getting out of it and doing very well. Now all those things have put a complexion on my life and the structure around it, which has always been difficult to deal with, but has been incredibly important in keeping me grounded in reality.

So for me it helps to explain why I feel relaxed at living in the East End and of working in a practice where communication, both within the practice team and with patients is so important, because that is what relationships are about for me. And I actually have no problem about living what people might call quite a 'low key' social life again because it fits with what I am, it fits with what I actually am involved in. And because my experience as a middle-class person has been so privileged into what working-class life ... living with someone who had that experience and being in contact with her parents and her sisters and all the rest of it.

... I don't know where it starts or comes from, but I think I have said again before that the key determinant of much of my emotional life must have been the death of my father when I was six. Now I can't remember ... OK fine, but that has been the pivotal event in my life in terms of, I can dump everything on – well of course my father died at six. Now that was a satisfactory, not satisfactory, that was a very unsatisfactory thing in my life in terms of understanding the implications for me and there is a recurrence several times through my life of going to people and saying – my father died when I was six, what effect do you think it has had on me? I have gone past that now to a stage where whatever effect it had on me I still have to make choices and decisions about my life and take responsibility for my own life. That transition happened around the time that I lived longer than he did i.e. when I was fifty.

... I was surrounded by women. My mother's sister, her husband died when I was about sort of three, so there was another single woman around. Two of their best friends who were around the house a bit as a child, were also widowed. There was my sister. The woman who was in effect, who I used to call my second mother, who was the woman who used to do the cleaning and the cooking and all that sort of stuff, ran the house really. She didn't live in, was a woman who was older than my mother, but was nevertheless a mother figure and a very significant mother figure in that sense. So I was a lone male, very much, from six until I went to university. In terms of getting involved with a working-class woman, I think, I feel very comfortable amongst working-class people. I just, I just think they are nearer to reality than middle-class people and I have that experience frequently. I am far more relaxed because there is a shared sort of vision of life that working-class people tend to have actually. I know other people deny this and it is classist and all the rest of it, but there is a 'them and us' understanding that working-class people are brought up with. For me I have met many that don't understand that. There are some right-wing working-class people but they still identify with the boss but understand the boss is different and for me to get involved with a working-class party ... and for me working-class life is the reality. Middle-class life is not the reality for me and you know people laugh about me not wearing a tie, or not doing this. I don't actually want to do that. It isn't natural in me to want to do it and I don't.

David shared deep uncertainties in our final interview:

I am wondering whether I am depressed or not and on balance I am probably not, but I haven't been, for instance, sleeping particularly well since August which is about the time when all the transition started. It is brand new for me, I have never not slept well before. And I am slightly worried about that, but then I think about the difficulties at home and the carrying of a partner who has been significantly depressed and I am sort of not surprised and I am reasonably happy to wait and see. I don't. I am not yet acting in a way that would worry me about being depressed but I do see Mary's psychiatrist with her at the same time. In fact we are going today. And he feels that I have been, quite naturally, under pressure from this and he also knows about the other work that I do. And it would quite easy, I have already had one conversation with him about me, it would be quite easy for me to see him about me specifically. So there is a lot of negative stuff around. But I am not panicking about it. I think that it will change and I am looking forward to the spring and summer really.

... So I would not take this to my own GP. It would be sort of pointless really. What is he going to say? I know what it is like. But then I tend to be, I monitor my own mental health quite well and quite objectively as much as anybody can. I tend not to panic. There are three or four around I could always just ring up if I just need to talk and I am feeling a bit miserable. And at the moment of course I have a direct line into the psychiatrist if I need one. I have been in therapy before. I could go back into therapy or I could chose some other ...

Well it is interesting. On the one hand Mary is preoccupied with herself and I was dealing with a lot of practice stuff in my holiday, which is not right. And the stuff about Trust and finances and the rest of it and Mary was completely brilliant. And she was interested in it but she was extremely good and helped me a lot to think through some of the issues ... But for most of the time the supportive side of our relationship is sort of fairly absent. And has been for a while, but there is not a lot I can do about that. And I think the depressing thing this time about her illness is that it is has been two years and is likely to be recurrent, certainly the anxiety, phobic side of it. And therefore I am sort of facing the prospect of life being, having that permanent level of difficulty. And it is an issue obviously.

... It makes me, the question I ask myself is, would she have been better if she had never met me? But I think that is a question that lots of people must ask each other in terms of relationships and I have sort of accepted that that is an irrelevant question because she did and we did and all the rest of it. I feel in some ways that I have brought problems to the relationship, but then again who wouldn't? The problems are circular. There are ways in which we have fed off each other's negative side in the same way as we have fed off each other's positive side. But that is life.

... I mean I have, I have a history of worrying or feeling, worrying about myself. I am not quite right. I ought to be feeling happier than I am. But that is a long-term thing. Chronic low-grade depression if you like. And I can remember in student days living in a house and a bloke who wasn't a medical student or anything, just a lodger, saying to me – your problem is that you are not happy unless you are worrying about something. Now it is often things like that which stick with you and someone said to me you seem very happy at the moment, you don't seem to be worrying at something. I said yes I am very worried about that. You know there is a way in which that is me gnawing away at whatever. And it is only over the last five years or so that I have come to terms with just accepting that is how I am in the same way that I will accept my mood going up and down and not expecting it to be terrible when I feel miserable, because that is pretty normal, but it bounces back.

We shared experience of psychotherapy as well as politics, of marriage as well as being driven as men. It was helpful, David said, to make these connections, 'therapeutic' even. It was the opportunity to talk in this way that was unusual. Doctors rarely did, except when forced into therapy themselves. I found it helpful too.

David talked about present fears.

I was talking to a mate last night who I meet regularly and although I wasn't talking about whether I was depressed or not I was talking about my future a lot and he is someone that often comes up with some very novel ideas and he did. And so that has sort of given me a bit of breathing space. But I am very watchful about myself at the moment. I think this is very significant stress I am under from various directions.

... And there aren't, yes there aren't other spaces to go to. You are probably right. So that is why it is all happening inside my head, because that is where it is taking place. There is nowhere else for it to take place. And I am only just becoming aware of these sorts of issues as we talk, because what you are saying is quite true. Fortunately although when you came in today it was a stressful environment I don't find the work that stressful. Even as I used to, say last year, because I was often rushing off to meetings. That is a great bonus that I can be here and not that stressed. I think stress is also, if I am more clear about what I am feeling … I am feeling that things are not right … I think I am reacting to a series of fairly major issues in my personal life, professionally and politically that I think are serious issues and will take a while to process.

We reviewed the research process, including the themes of gender and racism:

… society is both sexist and racist. And various attempts have been made to deal with that issue. It is therefore no surprise that the professions tend to follow that pattern. There has been an attempt, and it has only been a very weak attempt, to do something about that in terms of the medical profession. The issue for the medical profession is that, by and large, they deal with more women than men. And they deal with women, traditionally, incredibly badly … my politicisation began to take some sort of form in terms of my own actions, when a male gynaecologist got women to strip in front of the whole lot in order to do the examination. I witnessed that once, never again … the issue of gender is important in many ways but I don't see the medical profession doing an awful lot about it.

… medical culture is all about jokes and about humour and about, rather you know, awful attitudes to people …

And we returned to first impressions:

Well … it is not surprising that people perceive me as being hard, male aggressive, not aggressive, combative you know and therefore a million miles away from my feelings. I think that could be a character that people often see. It is played out in all sorts of ways you know. Don't approach David because he will just get angry or whatever. But because I don't feel a gulf between that, the positive side, the public side of me and where I live emotionally, because I don't feel the gulf, I assume that most people don't. But it is only when it is pointed out that I realise that I give off an air of being a million miles away from my emotions …

And all you can do, I think, is understand it enough in order to change your own personal behaviour.

... Well, we have travelled a long way. I mean when I talk about, as I did last night, explaining what you were doing I gave a précis on your work. There was this Tomlinson project and on the back of it you came along and evaluated what difference it made to how GPs learn and from that you began to hear things that set you along a particular way and that was about how professionals, GPs in this case, cope with all sorts of different aspects of their lives, including their personal. And therefore you found a way, some people have been nasty and say 'That is what sociologists do and the way they do it and that is why sociological theory is a nowhere sort of thing.' And other people have said 'Well that sounds a very serious approach to a complex issue' and I have certainly taken that view because I have found it useful to answer your questions – as so often happens when two people talk.

This has been therapeutic to me in the sense of having to piece together bits of it and come up with an answer. It is helpful because you are being challenged to make connections that you wouldn't normally do. So you can't avoid, in a sense, being therapeutic.

We had travelled a long way together in sharing stories, and in making connections between the inner and outer man, public personas and private selves. We promised to stay in touch to continue the conversation. He was unsure about next steps, but needed more support, and music. As for the GP role, being a businessman as well as a clinician, a manager as well as a reflective practitioner, was asking too much in the challenge of the inner-city, maybe more widely too. But then, as he spoke, he remembered particular Health Service managers and their behaviour. Blame, and not learning, was the culture; 'back to the politics, perhaps', David said, or was it to the gendered psychology of primary care, and of being a man?

13
Margins and Centres

The general point about the *contingency of the person* [original emphasis] – that being embedded in an environment, we are socially constructed beings – has led to the realisation that there is very little that is definitely fixed in the human sciences ... no fundamental and determining level in the psychological sphere ... no insulated gender essence.

Andrew Samuels, *The Political Psyche*

... Several features of the medical habitus may be at work to account for such high rates of many sorts of mental illness ... among members of the profession that itself treats illness ... the underlying importance of not complaining or 'whinging' ... the distaste for the low-Status segment of Psychiatry; unwillingness to examine, or unawareness of, internal mental events ... Perhaps the most important feature ... is the great difficulty doctors have in reversing their medical status and becoming a patient.

Simon Sinclair, *Making Doctors*

Introduction

This book has illuminated, in fine detail, how particular doctors respond to changing roles in a changing health-care system and society; and how this can be understood in a context of whole life histories and through the interpretive frame of a cultural psychology. Doctors, as a profession, have tended, for many reasons, to hide behind a professional curtain. The relationship, in particular, between their private selves and states, and those of their patients, has been a matter for discreet conversations behind closed doors. Some matters – surrounding the mental health of doctors – appear hard to talk about at all. There have been myriad surveys, of course, documenting the many problems of general practice and primary care in the inner-city, and measures taken of levels of distress among GPs, but relatively little has been heard from doctors themselves. This study has attempted to fill the gap, collaboratively, by creating space for them to tell their stories.

The twenty-five GPs cooperated, to varying extents, in drawing back the curtain on professional and personal dialectics, and on medicine and its mores. A conventional account of a doctor's work – and one doctors often themselves employ – is of a quasi-scientist, using well-tested procedures, based on the best evidence, in a highly rational, if also, it is admitted, on occasions, messy process. If the GP, compared to more specialist colleagues, adds a note on general practice being more down to earth and uncertain, the science and objectivity often remain central to the narrative. Moreover, getting on with the physical business of medicine in an objective way, and pushing the subjective and psychological to the margins, is often an implicit value within much of this lifeworld. It is a prejudice, and a set of priorities, which needs to be challenged.

This present study echoes many of Sinclair's findings, offering as it does complex insights into what can be a disturbing medical culture with its negative impact on the well-being of particular doctors. Medicine is a profession where it can be safer to pretend that all is well, even when palpably it is not. This is a world in which there is constant anxiety about what others might think and say in response to psychological distress. Yet, in the present study, there are also many heroic tales of GPs transcending the shortcomings of their professional world, and integrating subjective and psychological insight with medical and scientific knowledge, as well as cultural literacy, in a process of a profound lifelong learning, even if progress is often despite, rather than because of, the medical world they inhabit.

A starting point for the study was Berger and Mohr's account of the lifeworld of John Sassall, and how a doctor can feel haunted by the disturbance of others. There was also David Widgery's autobiography of being a GP in the East End of London which similarly captured feelings of impotence and despair in changing times. Such doctors may come to question their basic purpose, and the adequacy of their training and selves, when dealing with social pathologies and individual distress surrounding them. Such doctors can be driven over the edge. David Widgery was no exception among urban GPs; the present book has revealed the poor morale of many, the high levels of depression and stress, and how some have been close to the edge themselves. The evidence, when set alongside other studies, suggests a crisis, no less, for the profession and, by extension, our society. GPs are, whatever changes transpire in primary care, lynchpins of the health-care system: their well-being, the quality of their training and professional support and development structures matter.

The title of the book – *Doctors on the Edge* – represents, as the argument has evolved, an ambiguous metaphor of crisis but also opportunity. 'On the edge' suggests, of course, conditions of severe difficulty, of being pushed to extremes. But the metaphor can be read differently; as a cutting edge, as new forms of reflective practice where GPs are experimenting, eclectically, with diverse ways of working and learning about their role. And where learning about self, including from the patient within, is seen as essential to good practice and healthy development. The stories offer insights into what it takes – medically, psychologically, culturally, relationally and morally – to be an effective but also a realistic practitioner, and into the role of lifelong learning in the process. Such learning requires self-honesty and courage, as well as the support of others, and recognition too, lost in the omnipotent myth of some medicine, that taking care of a whole self is a prerequisite of taking care of whole others.

Threads

There are various threads connecting the stories together. The SDL movement represented a positive response to the crisis of caring and carers in inner-London. The groups were significant in providing a supportive space for many GPs to break free, for a while, from private fears and public personas, to share with colleagues the messiness, confusion, pain, vulnerability, as well as occasional exhilaration of the work. It was easier to talk there, given the groundrules and skilful facilitation. The impact of the groups varied, from individual to individual, although there was evidence, overall, that the groups contributed, via strengthened networks, to the establishment of more effective Primary Care Groups as well as boosting morale. Some people in the study were already engaged in extensive self-exploration and professional development of many kinds. Some understood the importance of understanding and transcending their own psychological pain, and of celebrating cultural 'otherness', in order to meet the needs of diverse patients. Some doctors, however, despite the best efforts of colleagues and health authorities to persuade them, avoided LIZEI more or less completely. The bitterness of some Asian doctors as to how they have been treated was intense.

Sarah Cotton and Ambi, in Chapter 5, illustrated the stresses of a particular day in June, and the range of problems – patient complaints, financial and business crises, abusive behaviour as well as family strains – which can beset the GP. This, in turn, raises questions about what is core, and what peripheral to the role. Being the businessperson, employer, manager and clinician may simply be too much. There are, it is to be noted, currently 300 pilot projects in 'Personal Medical Services' in England, where GPs are directly employed by Health Authorities rather than as independent contractors. One doctor in one pilot has stated: 'I can concentrate on the clinical side of things ... If I'd wanted to be a business man I'd have gone into business.' If the building is vandalised, on a run-down estate, the Health Authority pays (quoted in the *Guardian*, January 2000). Many of the doctors in this study would be horrified at such a development and the threat to their independence, real or imagined, but the issue of priorities needs to be addressed.

Aidene Croft and Daniel Cohen, because of gender, sexuality and/or wider life histories, took us into the creative edge of the profession. They were both outsiders within the 'malestream', and especially critical of their initial training and the wider culture of the profession. Health, for them, was part of a broad cultural, psychological and somatic canvas, in which many meanings could be found and a variety of approaches were needed. Daniel and Aidene used psychotherapy, as well as mature private relationships, in achieving levels of self-insight, and reflective practice, to better connect with their patients. The Somali refugee, despite the horrors inflicted on her family, personified a process in which a patient was treated as a whole being rather than pathologised. Talking of Darwin and adaptive skin conditions was the first time this patient had been taken seriously, treated humanely rather than as a one-dimensional 'problem'. It was Plato who said that we need the whole physician for the whole patient (Carmi, 2000). But the route to such wholeness can be, as McWhinney (1996) reminded us, long and tortuous, and the culture of silence that surrounds mental health inhibits many doctors from beginning the journey. Even those doctors with a deep commitment to Balint tend to hide core aspects of their identities in a culture in which the private and public have been kept firmly and unhealthily separate.

We came to understand, too, more of how particular GPs were haunted by unresolved issues from the past, and, at times, by overly omnipotent expectations of what they should expect of themselves, and of what others expected of them. Psychoanalytic ideas provide some possible insight in that Freud noted how the super-ego was deeply gendered, in effect, dependent on the child's relationship with the father. Crucially, to Freud, the super-ego was also the means by which culture obtained some mastery over id, over individual desire and aggression; over emotion, in other words (Connell, 1995). Medicine is, symbolically and emotionally, a patriarchal order where the word of an idealised and collective 'father' holds discursive sway. This is made manifest in the desire for order and detachment, for science and reason, in opposition to subjectivity, emotion and connectedness. What tends, too often, to be missing from the powerful collective myths of medicine is the need for 'parents' who are more flexible, who provide support and nurture, and who teach that emotion and shared responsibility are the routes to collective health.

The stories of Asian doctors, in Chapters 10 and 11, suggested a deeply unhealthy profession, with careers blighted by racism and the disdain of some colleagues. They were pilloried rather than supported for working on the margins, in the most deprived part of the inner-city. David Levine's story of a public man and his private pain, raised many questions including what may be required to support inner-city doctors and highlighted the need for a substantial investment in lifelong learning and more facilitative management. Managers could benefit from Balint or SDL groups too.

The shortcomings regarding initial training and continuing professional development of doctors are a central and persistent thread connecting all the stories. There were constant criticisms of overly textbook and factual approaches. For some, there was concern over medical reductionism as well as the racism and misogyny that infuse the training habitus. If the training was good for surgeons and other specialists, it was less so for those whose speciality was that of the generalist. While patients clearly want the most effective treatment available, based on the latest scientific evidence, it does not follow that most consultations require this. Rather, an empathic understanding of people and whole problems is what is most needed. Aidene Croft said she only really learned to be a GP after she left medical school. Daniel Cohen talked of the overt hostility of teachers and many students towards sociological and psychological insights. Medicine, and its training institutions, are revealed to be a culture in need of transformation. One solution might be for all trainee doctors to be attached, at an early and extensive stage, to general practice, rather than hospitals, to ground the medicine in wider social and personal awareness and encourage working in cooperation with a range of professionals.

A Cultural Psychology and Gender

Many gendered threads have been woven in the narrative. There is a devaluation of emotional labour both at work and in the home, and its psychological impact on women doctors – divided as they often are between the emotional demands of families and patients – can be considerable. The men, too often, tend to be too busy in their careers and emotionally absent, in certain respects at least, from the workplace and from home. Gender works at the mundane as well as the symbolic level. Stereotypical assumptions infuse the habits of mind and tacit everyday assumptions. These, in turn, are shaped by the insidious power of certain ideas within the culture, and, for that matter, the wider society.

Psychoanalysis can help explain how some of these processes work. For many feminist psychoanalysts, the main feature of their own and their mothers' socialisation, was the denial of women's own needs in preference to attending to the needs of others. Women have tended to be the midwives to others' desires (Schwartz, 1999). Women, in the main, in the surgery as elsewhere, provide the social lubricant to keep whole economies and societies moving. Jane Kelly's story, however, and others including Daniel Cohen's, offered glimpses of different possibilities in the new politics of identity, and of renegotiating relationships and their gendered assumptions, beyond the rigidities of social expectation and biological determinism. These stories also offered glimpses of new and more equitable divisions of labour that offer the possibility of new and diverse experiences for men and women alike, in medicine and the wider world, in private and public lives.

On Story, and Lifelong Learning

Stories, as anthropologists remind us, are the means by which humans make sense of experience. It may be a big story, such as science, or a more personal one, as we seek to make meaning, for instance, from birth or death or illness. The difficulty is that doctors have been taught to distrust their personal stories in the name of big science. Such science can be a normalizing truth that tends to disqualify, limit, deny or contain other potential stories (White and Epston, 1990). GPs are on the edge of the profession and its hierarchies of power and knowledge. Science has provided the discursive and bureaucratic base through which the medical profession has rationalised its privileged status in society but it has tended to marginalise other ways of knowing. What is suggested here is that doctors must find some means to weave more eclectic, personally authentic and experientially inclusive stories, using subjective/autobio-graphical understandings and psychological insights, alongside the science. If this is a hard road to travel, as McWhinney suggests, it is a necessary one for people dealing with the illness and dis-ease, in all its potential complexity, of others. It is, in the words of the Delors Report (1996) on lifelong learning, about learning how to be, to relate, to do as well as to think, in quite fundamental and challenging ways.

The problem is that of the profound split between personhood and medical practice; science from subjectivity in processes of healing and learning. Parker J. Palmer (1997) has observed that the split of the personal from academic practice is the consequence of a culture that distrusts the idea of personal truth. If the academy, including medicine, claims multiple ways of knowing a world, the objective way – taking us into 'the real world' and 'out of ourselves' – is a core value. The self within the culture is not a resource to be used but 'a danger to be suppressed, not a potential to be fulfilled but an obstacle to be overcome'. Palmer, because he is writing about education, refers to the need to recover the teacher within, the good object teacher we might have known as children, but tended to lose contact with on becoming an adult; someone who invites us to honour a truer self – not ego, expectations or image – but the core self. (I recognise the concept of the core self might raise major conceptual problems, associated as this is with the traditional liberal/humanist essentialist 'self'. This is not what I mean at all; rather I am thinking of the instinctual or primitive self, a self which has been taught, in earliest relationships – in the responses of the most significant others and in the mirroring of self in their eyes – either a sense of fundamental legitimacy and unconditional acceptance or their antithesis. In object relations theory, such a self is contingent on the other and developmental rather than a given.)

Note has been made, time and again, of how relations were at the heart of personal and professional development for many of the GPs. Significant others appear to be the key to risk taking, managing change and transition as well as professional development, in the broadest sense (Courtney, 1992; West, 1996). The good trainer, partner and/or colleague – when times are hard and the doctor feels inadequate – may be crucial to progress. Object relations theory offers a pragmatic perspective on the cultural psychology of such processes. The good object person can become available to us in later as well as early life, and can mirror other possibilities for a self in professional as well as personal life. The more we can people our minds with loving as well as diverse objects, and from a secure base of attachment, the more we are able to experiment with who and what we are, in healthy and psychologically progressive terms. Relationships are at the heart of professional and personal health as well as learning; they enable us to discover that we are, in the one person, many and varied people; and there are many and varied possibilities open to us. It was Freud who first suggested that humans were bisexual and that masculinity, like femininity, was precarious, complex and contingent. Self-composure, in the right context, can take many and diverse, rather than rigid and fixed, forms. There is in fact an important connection between the growing diversity of a postmodern culture and the potential diversity of selves, and learning, within it. Elena Michelson (1999) has written that the twentieth century was one in which various and vicious attempts have been made, by many groups and whole societies, to reject 'otherness'. Andrew Samuels (1993) has observed that cultural diversity and psychological plurality are no disaster but a challenge and opportunity to live fuller and more diverse lives.

Spirituality

There is another thread connecting the GPs' stories and spirituality. Andrew Samuels (1993) has drawn our attention to a growing 'resacralisation' in contemporary life, both in relationship to the natural world and in our relations with each other. Daniel Cohen and I considered spirituality in our conversations. He talked of the limits of knowing and of some of the mystery in the humanity that lies at the heart of a good doctor–patient relationship that cannot be reduced to a formula. He talked of 'spirit and God' as something we, in part, create. Julian Huxley (1957) considered us to be agents of the cosmos, helping it in some sense to know more of itself, that we may bear witness to its beauty, wonder and interest, and create something transcendental and life-enhancing in the process. Jung (1963) said that human beings cannot stand a meaningless existence. Harry Guntrip (1968), in exploring the connection between spirituality and inter-personal psychology, wrote that meaning and wholeness can finally only ever be constructed through our capacity for the personal life, which is always one of shared relationship. Maturity, and the construction of meaning and selfhood – a profoundly spiritual quest – is a steady enlarging of our scope for relating, first to those closest to us, and then on to difference, to wider communities and to humanity. There is a spiritual quest at the heart of becoming a doctor.

On Auto/biographical Research; and Narrative Truth

This research has worked from the premise that stories are never told in a vacuum, but are shaped in relationship with the researcher. Conventional distinctions between self and other, biography and autobiography, immediacy and memory disappear in this kind of participatory and collaborative work. The challenge was to create a method through which doctors were able, and secure enough, to talk openly and reflexively about their experience and life histories. Strong relationships were forged with particular doctors. These enabled me to better understand the workings of gender and cultural psychology across my own life; including in training to be a psychotherapist, as well as in the search to become a better partner and father. Some of the doctors taught me that if the 'feminine' has often been denied and split off in men's development and if masculinity has been constructed in overly aggressive and destructive terms, there is still a need, in each of us, men and women alike, to cultivate some 'masculine' traits. As Andrew Samuels (1993) has observed, we need power for subversion, a 'father-object' for breaking out, as well as preserving boundaries and one who enables the necessary subversion of older ways, but avoids being the overly reactionary parent who always says 'no'. A father-object who has remembered that always saying no, and being perpetually cautious, can mean psychological death. Doctors such as Daniel Cohen were in fact behaving like 'new men should', using power in life-enhancing ways, breaking prescriptions that can bind.

Such conclusions will no doubt evoke scepticism among readers trained in a more 'objective' and positivistic paradigm. They might also mention too that there are only twenty-five GPs in the study and the stories are probably unrepresentative of the wider profession. Large data sets and statistical relationships are at the core of conventional belief systems about what is good and rigorous research in medicine. It might also be suggested that the inner-city has more than its fair share of 'oddballs', professional 'down and outs' even, to make the study anything more than of particular interest. There is no convincing basis here from which to judge an entire profession. This takes us back to the question of validity. Jerome Bruner (1986) observed how the logico-scientific and narrative modes of thought differ in their approaches to this question. The former seeks to verify, by appeal to procedures, a formal and empirical truth; the other works towards verisimilitude, to the lifelikeness and meaningfulness of text. One works by reference to formal logic, tight analysis, empirical discovery, guided by reasoned hypotheses, and strives towards universal rather than particular truths, using, where possible, a mathematical system of description and explanation. The good story, on the other hand, gains its credence from engaging fully with the particulars of experience and from a process of transforming understanding in the generation of new insight and meaning. Validity lies in the quality of the process, the narrative truths generated, including their meaningfulness to others. Recovering in such detail – as these stories have – what is often silenced, as well as latent, in a doctor's life history, including the inter-subjectivity and pain at the heart of a doctor's work and learning, constitutes the good fiction and validity of this book. The abuse of power and status by some consultants, and the omnipotence rather than a sense of shared humanity that can haunt the profession, have been brought into sharper perspective as has the 'selective brain damage' of parts of initial training from which some GPs can take a lifetime to recover. And there is the story of the wounded or uncertain child within the doctor, who, lost and abandoned, has spent her time seeking to heal her world, and needs solace too, not the least from the parent that is the profession.

Baring souls in such ways, however, raised ethical questions. This was partly to do with an ever-present fear among some doctors of being recognised, and of careers being blighted as a result. Therefore transcripts were constantly revised and anonymised and the stories amended, at times substantially, without, it is hoped, jeopardising their narrative integrity. There is a further concern that such stories were so painful at times, that the boundary between research and therapy became problematic. But even if the boundary was difficult, many of the GPs welcomed the opportunity to speak openly and reflexively about their lives and roles, often for the first time, and felt better for it. It was not 'the norm' to talk, and share in such ways.

Some doctors were close to the edge, which worried me. John Sassall's suicide came to mind and I wondered about the effect on him of Berger's *A Fortunate Man*. I wrote to John Berger and he sent me the draft of a postscript to a recently published German edition of the book:

When I wrote the preceding pages – and I'm thinking particularly of the last ones which speak of the impossibility of summing up Sassall's life and work – I did not know that years later he was going to shoot himself.

Our instant-hedonist culture tends to believe that a deliberate suicide is a negative comment. What went wrong? It naively asks. Yet a suicide does not necessarily constitute a criticism of the life being ended, it may belong to that life's destiny. This was the tragic Greek view.

John the man I loved killed himself. And, yes, his death has changed the story of his life. It has made it more mysterious. Not darker. I see as much light there as ever. Simply more mysterious. This mystery makes me feel more modest, as I stand before him. And standing before him, I do not search for what I might have foreseen and didn't – as if the essential was missing from what passed between us; rather I now begin with his violent death, and, from it, look back with increased tenderness on what he set out to do and what he offered to others, for as long as he could endure.

I grew close to certain doctors in this present project and worried about them and the impact of the research on their condition. I became more aware too, of the impact of an inner-city's disturbance on committed, caring people. Suicide has meaning, and Berger, echoing the Greeks, is right in this. But suicide can be a waste too, and unnecessary. The feelings of desperation and distress of many doctors can be understood and responded to differently, in terms of a profession that needs, emotionally, to grow up, and where varied meanings can be found by transcending disturbance in different ways, via the support and care of others; and that has learned, somewhat better, to share many stories, more openly. Daniel Cohen, David Levine and others consistently said, when asked about the process, 'I am doing this for my benefit too.' Far more spaces are needed where doctors can, imaginatively and collaboratively, generate stories together.

A Conclusion, and Beginning?

How do we conclude such a story, given that the process is never complete and experience is always provisional? Doctors have to learn, as we all do, how to live in perpetual transition. Life is not predictable and we have to remain open, flexible and resilient – rather than defensive and paranoid – in the face of change. But the creative world can also be playful, as Wheatley and Kellner-Rogers(1996) have written in considering what they term a new science. They point the way to the openness and flexibility we require to be lifelong learners. Such a message is bigger than individuals. None of us, in the final resort, needs to struggle to create ourselves in isolation. Every change we make in ourselves, every exploratory path we follow, changes many others. Our explorations may even change the rules by which we change. We are not, inevitably and forever, contestants pitted against one another in a game with all the rules set ahead of time. The world is potentially more playful, and transformational, than this. Life invites us to create not only the forms but also the processes of discovery. That invitation is at the heart of healing too.

Of course there may, in a postmodern spirit, be more pessimistic readings of the doctors' texts, and of the possibilities for transforming the profession and health care. Some doctors were feeling deeply depressed at what was happening to their role. If patients were demanding, in effect, more holistic sensitivities, there were powerful forces pulling in opposite directions. Christopher Lasch (1995) has written, in an American context, about the conflict between broader and narrower constructs of psychological medicine. Freud's vision, he argues, was of psychological processes encouraging introspection, and aiming at the development of moral insight. But this humane and meaning-making vision may be under threat from a 'quick fix', consumerist mentality, using drugs and behaviour modification. It is interesting that a recent report on primary care, from a NHS-user survey, suggested that patients place greater value on easy access to care than a long-term relationship with their personal doctor (the *Guardian*, 2000). Yet, as three GPs have reminded us (Dixon, Sweeney and Pereira Gray, 1999), the physician as healer, as well as scientist, 'is now poised to rise again like the phoenix'. Because, as they put it, 'modern science demands it'. The modern GP needs to fill the gap left by the very impersonality of modern science.

The quality of the relationship between therapist and patient – what is often termed the working alliance – is central to effective psychological care. Alan Cartwright (1999), a psychotherapist and researcher, wrote that the composite image of the good therapist, from the viewpoint of patients, was the keenly attentive, interested, benign, good listener. Someone who is a friend and who is warm and natural and does not shrink from giving direct advice. A person, too, who speaks an intelligible language. Millions of pounds, he suggests, have been spent trying to demonstrate that the outcome of therapy is the result of some special technical expertise or theory, but this has not been a successful venture: 'I have come to the conclusion that all the technical expertise of the therapist has to be expressed in such a framework ... an ability to remain therapeutic when others would become persecutory and all of the theories become condensed into the ability to comprehend that which seems incomprehensible and to express that understanding by making the right remark at the right time.' Such an observation could apply, to a large extent, to general practice. The ability to comprehend what may seem incomprehensible, and to express an understanding through the right remark, is no simple matter of chance or communication skill, to be taught in a month's module. Rather it is a consequence of a lifetime's courageous learning, one shaped and shared in relationship, against a backcloth of a culture only gradually becoming more conscious of itself and its gendered constraints and possibilities.

APPENDIX

General Practitioners, Learning and Health Care in the Inner-City

**A Study Being Undertaken by Linden West
at the University of Kent**

Notes of Guidance for Interviewees and Conditions of Use Form

1. This particular research project is concerned to understand processes of health care, in the context of a changing health service as well as change in professional and wider socio-cultural contexts. It focuses on health care in the inner-city and the role of education, and other factors, for better and worse, in the management of change. The biographical methodology involves conducting a series of interviews over a period of time with a view to understanding experiences in the total context of a person's life history and current circumstances.

2. Interviews are being conducted with twenty-five General Practitioners from a number of inner-city locations.

3. Given the potentially sensitive nature of the material you have an absolute right to refuse to answer any questions asked as well as to withdraw from the research at any stage. I will be careful not to push you in directions you do not wish to go, or to assume the role of the therapist.

4. You have the right to withdraw retrospectively any consent given and to require that your data, including recordings, be destroyed. Obviously, it is important for the researchers to know your position as soon as possible after reading transcripts. Refusal or withdrawal of consent would normally therefore be within two weeks of receiving a copy of the transcript.

5. Confidentiality is a key issue. I will provide each interviewee with a Conditions of Use form which will allow you to preserve anonymity if you

so wish. As a general rule the material is to be used for research purposes only (unless prior permission has been obtained, for example to use tapes in teaching). I will take all steps, if this is what you desire, to preserve your anonymity in the presentation of case studies.

6. Each of you will be given transcripts of your interviews and, if you wish, a copy of your tapes. You may edit the transcript as you see fit and we would like you to return the final form of all transcripts two months after receipt of the final one. The final edited versions of the transcripts and all the tapes will be kept with the researcher (Linden West) in the university. Apart from the specified researcher any other access will be with your permission only.

7. In general terms these procedures are informed by the British Psychological Society's Statement of Ethical Principles which are set out in the January 1993 edition of *The Psychologist*.

8. Thank you for all your help in and contribution to the research.

General Practitioners, Health and Learning in the Inner-City

Conditions of Use Form

1. I agree to the material on tape and transcript being used for research purposes as part of the above project, subject to the conditions specified in the Notes of Guidance attached to this form. I understand access to it is restricted to Linden West, unless specific, additional agreement is obtained.

2. I request/do not request (delete as appropriate) that my anonymity is preserved in the use of the material via the use of pseudonyms etc.

3. Any other comments

Signed

Name (please print)

Address and telephone number

Date

Time Line/Fact Sheet

Name, address, telephone number

Date of birth

Place of birth

Current role, nature of practice: i.e. group, fund-holding, staffing etc.

Family of origin: mother and father, occupations, siblings etc.

Schooling/education, with dates and locations

Professional training, with dates and location

Qualifications, with dates

Significant continuing education experiences, details with dates

Details of medical career (and other careers, where relevant) with dates

Professional activities, membership of professional bodies, involvement therein, with dates

Significant professional/career events, other than those above, with details and dates

Any other relevant career or related information

Bibliography

AGIY/FIS (1997) *Meeting Diverse Needs*. London: Action Group for Action Youth and Federation of Irish Societies.

Arendt, H. (1998) *The Human Condition*. Chicago: University of Chicago Press.

Balint, E., Courtenay, M., Elder, A., Hull, S. and Julian, P. (1993) *The Doctor, the Patient and the Group*. London: Routledge.

Balint, M. (1957) *The Doctor, his Patient and the Illness*. London: Pitman Paperbacks.

Bardsley, M., Barker, M., Bhan, A., Farrow, S., Gill, M., Jacobson, B. and Morgan, D. (1998) *Health of Londoners, a Public Health Report for Londoners*. London: Kings Fund.

Bennett. C. (1998) 'Dirty Doctors' in the *Guardian*. 21 December, 25.

Bennet, G. (1998) 'The Doctor's Losses: Ideals Versus Realities' in *BMJ*. Vol. 316, 18 April, 1238–40.

Berger, J. and Mohr, J. (1967) *A Fortunate Man, The Story of a Country Doctor*. London: Writers and Readers Co-op.

Brindle, D. (2000) 'Healthy Side-effects of Bypassing the Rule Book' in the *Guardian*, 6 January, 8.

Bruner, E. (1986) 'Experience and its Expressions', in Turner, V. and Bruner, E. (eds), *The Anthropology of Experience*. Chicago: University of Illinois Press.

Bruner, J. (1986) *Actual Minds, Possible Worlds*. Cambridge, Mass.: Harvard University Press.

Bruner, J. (1990) *Acts of Meaning*. Cambridge, Mass.: Harvard.

Buber, M. (1965) *The Knowledge of Man*. New York: HarperCollins.

Burton, J. (1997) 'An Approach to Evidence-based Medicine', Paper to the IERG. Cambridge.

Burton, J. (1998) Private Communication.

Burton, J. (2000), Private Communication.

Byatt, A.S. and Sodre, I. (1995) *Imagining Characters, Six Conversations about Women Writers*. London: Chatto and Windus.

Cape, J. (1996) 'Psychological Treatment of Emotional Problems by General Practitioners' in *British Journal of Medical Psychology 69*. (5), 85–9.

Carmi, M. (2000) 'Mystery in Medicine and Education: A Journey from General Practice to Primary Care', Professorial Lecture. University of Middlesex, January.

Carmi, M. and Hiew, S. (1997) 'Self-Directed Learning Groups', Paper to the IERG. Cambridge.

Cartwright, A. (1999) 'Thoughts on Retiring as Director of the Centre for the Study of Psychotherapy', Paper to the Canterbury Consortium of Psychoanalytic Psychotherapists.

Clarke, M. (2000) Private Communication.

Clough, P. (1996) 'Again Fathers and Sons: The Mutual Construction of Self, Story and Special Educational Needs', *Disability and Society, 11* (1), 71–81.

Cochrane, R. and Singh, S. (1989) 'Mental Hospital Admission Rates of Immigrants to England: a Comparison of 1971 and 1981' in *Social Psychiatry and Psychiatric Epidemiology 24*, 2-11.

Commission on Social Justice (1994) *Social Justice: Strategies for National Renewal.* London: Vintage.

Connell, R.W. (1995) *Masculinities.* London: Polity Press.

Courtney, S. (1992) *Why Adults Learn: Towards a Theory of Participation in Adult Education.* London: Routledge.

Delors, J (1996) *Learning: The Treasure Within.* Paris: UNESCO.

Dennick, R. and Exley, K. (1998) 'Radical Changes in Medical Culture' in *The New Academic.* Summer, London, 17–19.

Department of Health (1998) *Our Healthier Nation.* London: The Stationery Office.

Dixon, D., Sweeney, K. and Pereira Gray, D. (1999) 'The Physician Healer: Ancient Magic or Modern Science?' *British Journal of General Practice.* April, 309–12.

Donne, J., 'Satyre 111' in Grierson, H. (1971) *Donne, Poetical Works.* Oxford: University Press.

Ecclestone, K. (1996) 'The Reflective Practitioner; Mantra or Model for Emancipation?' in *Studies in the Education of Adults.* 28 (2) 146–61.

Edwards, P. and Flatley, J. (1996) (eds) *The Capital Divided: Mapping Poverty and Social Exclusion in London.* London: London Research Centre.

Elder, A. (1999) 'Thoughts From the Front-line, Why Balint Still Matters', Paper to a Conference, Learning the Reality of Primary Care. Tavistock Clinic/Regional GP Postgraduate Deanery, March.

Evans, M. (1993) 'How the Personal Might be Social', in *Sociology, 27* (1) 5–14.

Fine, M. (1992) 'Passions, Politics and Power' in Fine, M. (ed.) *Disruptive Voices, the Possibilities of Feminist Research.* 205–31.

Forna, A. (1999) *Mother of all Myths; How Society Moulds and Constrains Mothers.* London: HarperCollins.

Foucault, M. (1979) *Discipline and Punish: The Birth of the Prison.* London: Allen Lane.

Frosh, S. (1991) *Identity Crisis: Modernity, Psychoanalysis and the Self.* London: Macmillan.

Frosh, S. (1994) *Sexual Difference; Masculinity and Psychoanalysis.* London: Routledge.

Gay, P. (1988) *Freud, A Life for Our Time.* London: Macmillan.

Giddens, A. (1991) *Modernity and Self Identity; Self and Society in the Late Modern Age.* London: Polity.

Glaser, D. and Frosh, S. (1988) *Child Sexual Abuse.* London: Macmillan.

Greenhalgh, T. (1998) 'Narrative Based Medicine in an Evidence Based World' in Greenhalgh, T. and Hurwitz, B. (eds) *Narrative Based Medicine, Dialogue and Discourse in Clinical Practice.* London: BMJ, 247–65.

Greenhalgh, T. and Hurwitz, B. (1998) *Narrative Based Medicine, Dialogue and Discourse in Clinical Practice.* London: BMJ.

Guntrip, H. (1968) 'Psychology and Spirituality', in James, E. (ed.) *Spirituality for Today.* London: SCM Press, 87–102.

Hall, S. (1992) 'New Ethnicities' in Donald, J. and Rattansi, A. (eds) *Race, Culture and Difference.* 252–59.

Haraway, D. (1988) 'Situated Knowledges: The Science Question in Feminism and the Privilege of the Partial Perspective', in *Feminist Studies.* 14, 575–99.

Hardy, T. (1902) 'De Profundis' in *Collected Poems of Thomas Hardy.* London: Macmillan.

Harrison, J. and West, L. (1997) 'Telling Stories, Self-Directed Learning, General Practice and the Inner-City', Paper to the IERG Group.

Harrison, R. (1997) *Guidance in Context, the Role of Guidance in an Employee Development Scheme.* Milton Keynes: Open University.

Hart, M. (1998) 'The Experience of Living and Learning in Different Worlds' in *Studies in Continuing Education.* 20 (2), 187–200.

Heath, I. (1998) 'Following the Story; Continuity of Care in General Practice', in Greenhalgh, T. and Hurwitz, B. (eds) *Narrative Based Medicine.* London: *BMJ*, 83–92.

Henley, P. (1997) 'The Teller, the Tale and the Tape', in the *Times Literary Supplement.* 6–8.

Hey, A. (1999) 'Troubling the Auto/Biography of the Questions: Re/thinking Rapport and the Politics of Social Class in Feminist Participant Observation', Paper to the Second International Conference, Gender and Education. Warwick, March.

Hodgkin, P. (1996) 'Medicine, Postmodernism, and the End of Certainty,' *BMJ* Editorial, No. 7072, 21–28 December.

Holmes, J. (1996) *John Bowlby and Attachment Theory.* London: Routledge.

Holmes, J. (1998) 'The Changing Aims of Psychoanalytic Psychotherapy, An Integrative Perspective', in the *International Journal of Psychoanalysis.* 79, 227–40.

Humphries, S. (1984) *The Handbook of Oral History, Recording Life Stories.* London, Inter-Action.

Hutton, W. (1995) *The State We're In.* London: Jonathan Cape.

Huxley, J. (1957) *New Bottles for New Wine.* London: Harper Row.

Ingleby, D. (1998) 'Culture and Medical Health, A Radical Agenda', The Tizard Centre Open Lecture. University of Kent, Canterbury, 11 December.

Inglis, F. (1995), *Raymond Williams.* London: Routledge.

Jain, A. and Ogden, J. (1999) 'General Practitioners' Experiences of Patients' Complaints: Qualitative Study', *BMJ*, 318, 1596–99.

Josselson, R. and Lieblich, A. (1995) *The Narrative Study of Lives.* London: Sage.

Jung, C.G. (1963) *Memories, Dreams, Reflections.* London: Collins.

Kleinman, A. and Cohen, A. (1997) 'Psychiatry's Global Challenge' in *Scientific American.* March, 74–7.

Lasch, C. (1995) *The Revolt of the Elites and the Betrayal of Democracy.* New York: Norton and Company.

Launer, J. (1996) 'An Education in the Art of Effective Tuition' in *Doctor,* 11 January 42–3.

Launer, J. (1998) 'Narrative and Mental Health in Primary Care' in Greenhalgh, T. and Hurwitz, B. (eds) *Narrative Based Medicine.* 93–102.

Llewelyn, S. and Osborn, K. (1990) *Women's Lives,* London: Routledge.

London AUDGP Group (1997) Addressing the Urban Dimension in General Practice, Annual Scientific Meeting. Madingley, Cambridge, February.

Main, T. (1978) 'Some Medical Defences Against Involvement with Patients, Michael Balint Memorial Lecture', *Journal of Balint Society.* January, 3–11.

Mann, S. and Pedler, M. (1992) (Guest eds), 'Biography in Management and Organisational Development', *Management Education and Development.* 23 (3) London.

McBride, M. and Metcalfe, D. (1995) 'General Practitioners' Low Morale: Reasons and Solutions' in *British Journal of General Practice.* May, 227–9.

McWhinney, I. (1996) 'The Importance of Being Different; the William Pickles Lecture', *British Journal of General Practice.* 46, 433–6.

Miller, N. (1993) *Personal Experience, Adult Learning and Social Research.* Centre for Research in Adult Education for Human Development, University of South Australia.

Michelson, E. (1999) 'Carnival, Paranoia and Experiential Learning' in *Studies in the Education of Adults.* Vol. 31 (2), 140–54.

Miller, N. and West, L. (1998) 'Connecting the Personal and the Social', in *Research, Teaching and Learning, Proceedings of the 28th Annual Conference, SCUTREA.* Exeter, July, 163–8.

Mitchell, J. (1974) *Psychoanalysis and Feminism.* London: Harmondsworth/Penguin.

Morris, P. (1998) Paper to the IERG. Cambridge.

Newman, J. (1999) 'Gender and Cultural Change' in *Gender, Culture and Organisational Change, Putting Theory into Practice.* London: Routledge 11–29.

NHS Executive (1998) *Development through Education, the Lessons of the LIZEI for Primary Care.* London: Department of Health.

Palmer, P.J. (1997) 'The Heart of the Teacher; Identity and Integrity in Teaching' in *Change.* November/December, 15–21.

Parsons, C. (1999) *School Exclusions.* London: Routledge.

Peters, T. and Waterman, R. (1995) *In Search of Excellence.* London: HarperCollins.

Pietroni, R. (1992) 'New Strategies for Higher Professional Education', in *British Journal of General Practice.* Vol. 42, 294–6.

Polanyi, L. (1985) *Telling the American Story: A Structural and Cultural Analysis of Conversational Storytelling.* Norwood, NJ: Ablex.

Randall, W. (1995) *The Stories We Are; An Essay in Self-Creation.* Toronto, University Press.

Reid, M. (1982) 'Marginal Man: The Identity Dilemma of the Academic General Practitioner', *Symbolic Interaction,* 5, 325–42.

Reiss, M. (1997) 'Is Your Doctor a Good Communicator?' *Paper to the IERG.* Cambridge.

Rich (1972) 'When We Dead Awaken. Writing as Revision', *College English* 34(1), 18–25.

Ross, F. and Meerabeau, L. (1997) Editorial, *Journal of Interprofessional Practice,* 11(1), April.

Rout, U. (1996) 'Stress Among General Practitioners and their Spouses: a Qualitative Study' in *British Journal of General Practice.* March, 157–60.

Royal College of General Practitioners (1993), *Stress Management in General Practice, Report of the RCGP Stress Management Working Party,* Occasional Paper 61.

Royal College of General Practitioners (1994) *Report of the Inner-City Task Force.* Occasional Paper 66.

Sackett, D., Rosenburg, W. and Hayes, R. (1997) *Evidence-Based Medicine, How to Practice and Teach EBM.* New York: Churchill Livingstone.

Sackin, P. (1994) 'What is a Balint-group?' in *Journal of the Balint Society.* 22, 36–7.

Samuels, A. (1985) *Jung and the Post-Jungians.* London: Routledge.

Samuels, A. (1993) *The Political Psyche.* London: Routledge.

Savage, R. (1991) 'Continuing Education for General Practice: A Lifelong Journey', Editorial, *British Journal of General Practice,* 41, 311–14.

Sayers, J. (1995) *The Man Who Never Was, Freudian Tales.* London: Chatto and Windus.

Schmitt, R. (1996) 'Racism and Objectification: Reflections on Themes from Fanon' in Lewis, R., Gordon, T., Denlan Sharpley-Whiting, T. and White, R. (eds) *Fanon: a Critical Reader*. Oxford: Blackwell, 35–50.

Schon, D. (1987) *Educating the Reflective Practitioner*. San Francisco: Jossey-Bass.

Schwartz, J. (1999) *Cassandra's Daughter; A History of Psychoanalysis in Europe and America*. London: Allen Lane.

Seidler, V. (1994) *Unreasonable Men; Masculinity and Social Theory*. London: Routledge.

Sinclair, S. (1997) *Making Doctors*. Oxford: Berg.

Spender, D. (1981) 'The Patriarchal Paradigm and the Response to Feminism' in Spender, D. (ed.), *Men's Studies Modified, the Impact of Feminism on Academic Disciplines*. Oxford: Pergamon Press, 155–74.

Stanley, I., Al-Shehri, A. and Thomas, P. (1993) 'Continuing Education for General Practice, 1. Experience, Practice and the Media of Self-directed Learning for Established General Practitioners', in *British Journal of General Practice*, 43, 210–14.

Stanley, L. (1994) *The Auto/biographical I*. Manchester: University Press.

Symonds, A. (1979) 'The Wife as the Professional' in *The American Journal of Psychoanalysis 39*, 55–63.

The Turnberg Report (1997); Royal College of Physicians of London, *Improving Communication between Doctors and Patients – A Report of a Working Party*. London.

Tilki, M. (1996) 'The Health of the Irish in Britain', *Federation of Irish Studies Bulletin*. 9, 11–14.

Tomlinson, Sir Bernard (1992); *Report of the Committee of Enquiry into London's Health Service, Medical Education and Research*. London: HMSO.

Thomson, A. (1994) *Anzac Memories*. Auckland: Oxford University Press.

Thomson, E. (1963) *The Making of the English Working Class*. London: Penguin.

Townsend, D., Davidson, N. and Whitehead, M. (1992) *Inequalities in Health*. London: Penguin (containing the Black Report and the Health Divide).

Viney, L. (1993) *Life Stories; Personal Construct Therapy with the Elderly*. Chichester: John Wiley and Sons.

Ward, K. (1995) 'Community Regeneration and Social Exclusion', Paper to the Universities Association for Continuing Education. April, Swansea.

Webster, C. (1998) *The National Health Service, a Political History*. Oxford: OUP.

West, L. (1996) *Beyond Fragments, Adults, Motivation and Higher Education; A Biographical Analysis*. London: Taylor and Francis.

West, L. (1999) 'Gendered Transitions', Paper to the ESREA Gender Network Conference. April, Bochum.

Wheatley, M. and Kellner-Rogers, M. (1996) *A Simpler Way*. San Francisco: Berrett-Koehler.

White, M. and Epston, D. (1990) *Narrative Means to Therapeutic Ends*. London: Norton.

Whitehead, S. (1997) 'The Gendered Transition of Educational Management', Paper to the Gender and Educational International Conference. Warwick, April.

Widgery, D. (1993) *Some Lives, A GP's East End*. London: Simon and Schuster.

Index

Compiled by Sue Carlton